INTERMITTENT FASTING FOR WOMEN OVER 40

A SIMPLE GUIDE TO SHED BELLY FAT, BALANCE HORMONES, UNLOCK HEALTHY AGING, AND BOOST ENERGY FOR A HEALTHIER YOU

INFINITE HEALTH PUBLISHING

Copyright © 2025 by Sunflower Publishing Creations LLC

All rights reserved.

The content within this book may not be reproduced, duplicated or transmitted without direct written permission from the author or the publisher.

Under no circumstances will any blame or legal responsibility be held against the publisher, or author, for any damages, reparation, or monetary loss due to the information contained within this book. Either directly or indirectly. You are responsible for your own choices, actions, and results.

Legal Notice

This book is copyright protected. This book is only for personal use. You cannot amend, distribute, sell, use, quote or paraphrase any part, of the content within this book, without the consent of the author or publisher.

Disclaimer Notice

Please note the information contained within this document is for educational and entertainment purposes only. All effort has been expended to present accurate, up-to-date, and reliable, complete information. No warranties of any kind are declared or implied. Readers acknowledge that the author is not engaging in the rendering of legal, financial, medical or professional advice. The content within this book has been derived from various sources. Please consult a licensed professional before attempting any techniques outlined in this book.

By reading this document, the reader agrees that under no circumstances is the author responsible for any losses, direct or indirect, which are incurred as a result of the use of the information contained within this document, including, but not limited to, — errors, omissions, or inaccuracies.

CONTENTS

Introduction — v

Chapter 1 — 1
Intermittent Fasting and Hormonal Health

Chapter 2 — 20
Cycle-Specific Fasting

Chapter 3 — 33
Nutritional Foundations for Successful Fasting

Chapter 4 — 47
Enhancing Energy and Mental Clarity

Chapter 5 — 62
Sustainable Weight Management and Symptom Relief

Chapter 6 — 75
Longevity and Disease Prevention

Chapter 7 — 88
Interactive Elements and Personalized Fasting Journeys

Chapter 8 — 104
Integrating Fasting Into Everyday Life

Conclusion — 117

Bibliography — 123

INTRODUCTION

"The greatest revolution of our generation is the discovery that human beings can alter the quality of their lives by altering the attitudes of their minds." — Albert Schweitzer

I stood in front of the mirror, feeling like a stranger in my own skin. My energy levels were low, my mood was unpredictable, and no matter what I ate or how much I exercised, that stubborn belly fat refused to budge. I was in my forties, and my body had started writing its own rules. Initially, I chalked it up to having a baby at thirty-nine. I had heard that your body doesn't recover quite so quickly. But as I approached forty-five, I knew I needed a change—not just a quick fix but a practical and maintainable way to reclaim my health and energy.

That's when I stumbled upon intermittent fasting. Initially, I was skeptical. Could it really help with the challenges of being over forty, especially with the whirlwind of hormonal changes I was experiencing? But I was willing to try. What I found was not just a method for weight management but a transformative approach aligned with my body's natural rhythms.

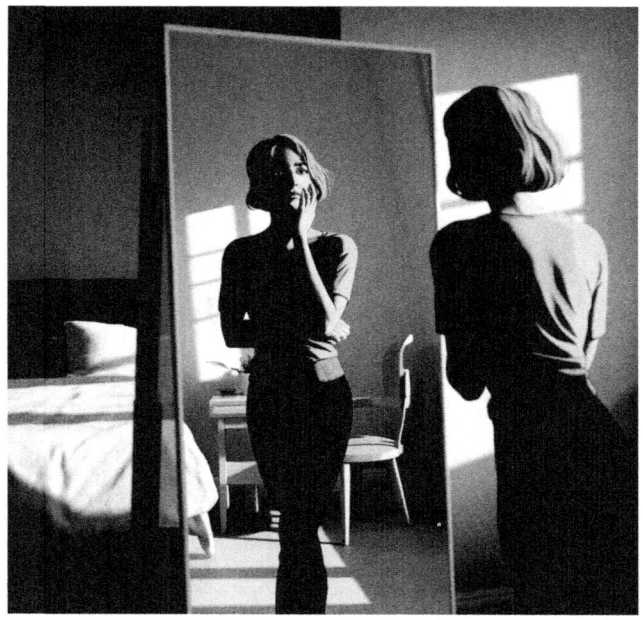

My own transformation through intermittent fasting surprised even me. Within the first month, I noticed I was no longer reaching for that three p.m. coffee just to get through the day. The brain fog that had become my constant companion started lifting, and I found myself thinking more clearly during morning meetings. By month three, my clothes fit differently—and they weren't just looser. I was carrying myself with more confidence.

And the most unexpected change?

My sleep improved dramatically. No more tossing and turning or middle-of-the-night anxiety. But perhaps the most meaningful change was that I finally felt in control of my health again. Gone were the days of feeling helpless about my expanding waistline or unpredictable energy levels. Plus, these weren't just temporary fixes. They were sustainable improvements that made me feel like myself again—just better.

Women over forty face many unique challenges. Hormonal shifts during perimenopause and menopause, and then after menopause, can lead to weight gain, fatigue, and mood swings. These years can feel like an uphill battle as we try to maintain the energy and health we once took for granted. Your confidence takes a hit, and you can't shake the frustration.

I looked for answers to the whys, but all the resources I found fell short. The lack of information and support motivated me to write this book. As I learned more about the science and had my own successes, I felt even more driven to tell this story and offer empowering solutions to others. This book is designed specifically with you in mind. I want to help you navigate intermittent fasting in a way that respects and supports the changes your body is undergoing.

Scientific research supports intermittent fasting's numerous benefits. It can:

- Help manage weight
- Balance hormones
- Increase energy
- Unlock healthy aging

The idea is simple: Give your body regular breaks from digestion, allowing it to use energy more efficiently and reset its metabolic processes.

There are many misconceptions about fasting, especially for women in our age group. I've heard them all. Some believe it might not work with their schedules or that it could disrupt their already fluctuating hormones. Others think they will need to skip meals or starve themselves.

One of the biggest concerns I hear is, "Won't I be hungry all the time?" I had the same worry when I started. But here's what surprised me and what research confirms: Our bodies are remarkably adaptable. Within just a few weeks of starting intermittent fasting, most women find their hunger patterns shift naturally. You'll discover that true hunger is different from habitual eating, and you'll develop a new awareness of your body's signals. Many women in our program actually report feeling less hungry overall, with more stable energy throughout the day.

Remember, this isn't about starving yourself. It's about finding your body's natural rhythm and working with it, not against it. However, the consensus of clinicians and dieticians shows that intermittent fasting can be a powerful tool for women over forty when done mindfully. It's about finding the right balance and listening to what your body needs. Fasting may seem a bit scary at first, but once you hear about its benefits and flexibility, you will see that it is a very simple and easy way to take control of your health and wellness.

You might be wondering how long it takes to see and feel results with intermittent fasting. While every woman's journey is unique, most of the women I've worked with notice subtle changes within the first two weeks—often starting with improved mental clarity and better sleep. By week three or four, many report more stable energy levels and fewer cravings. Physical changes, like improvements in body composition, typically become noticeable around six to eight weeks.

But here's what I want to emphasize: This isn't a race. Some women adapt quickly, while others need more time to find their rhythm. The key is to be patient with yourself and celebrate the small victories along the way. Remember, we're not just looking for quick results. We're creating sustainable habits that will serve us well into our fifties and beyond.

In this book, we'll take a systematic journey through everything you need to know about intermittent fasting for our age group. You'll start by understanding how fasting works with your hormones, not against them, and explore how to adapt your fasting schedule to your natural cycles. You'll learn the nutritional foundations that make fasting both effective and enjoyable and discover how to boost your energy and mental clarity along the way.

Then you'll tackle the practical aspects of weight management and symptom relief, while looking ahead to the powerful long-term benefits for healthy aging and disease prevention. The final chapters will help you create your own personalized fasting approach and seamlessly integrate it into your daily life, complete with interactive tools and trackers to support your journey.

Each chapter builds upon the last, giving you a comprehensive understanding while keeping things practical and actionable.

I know many of us are the heart of our families and social circles—planning meals, organizing gatherings, and juggling countless responsibilities. One of the most common concerns I hear is, "How will I handle family dinners or social events while fasting?" The beauty of intermittent fasting is its flexibility. You'll learn how to adjust your fasting windows to accommodate family mealtimes, special occasions, and social commitments. Many women in our community have found creative ways to make it work, from scheduling their eating window around family dinnertime to adapting their fasting schedule for weekend brunches with friends. Your family can even become your biggest supporters once they see how energized and happy you become.

Remember, this journey isn't about isolation or missing out on life's important moments. It's about finding a sustainable rhythm that enhances both your health and your relationships.

This book is more than just a guide. It's an invitation to join a community of women on the same journey. You'll find stories and testimonials from others who have successfully integrated intermittent fasting into their lives. And remember, you are not alone in this. Together, we can share experiences, support each other, and celebrate our successes.

As you read, expect to find actionable tips, meal plans, and interactive elements, like fasting trackers, to help you track your progress. We'll explore practical strategies that fit your lifestyle so that this journey is manageable and rewarding. I'll share some success stories from women who have been where you are now, which will inspire and motivate you.

I am passionate about intermittent fasting because it has improved my life tremendously. Now it's my time to pay it forward and share this knowledge and experience to help you overcome the challenges I've faced and overcome and achieve a healthier, more energetic life. While I'm not a physician or nutritionist, my approach to intermittent fasting is rooted in evidence-based strategies that consider the unique needs of women in these transformative years.

I was lucky enough to have a physician and nutritionist who both supported intermittent fasting and helped me with a personalized plan that has worked for me over the years. This book will cover tools you can use to develop your own personalized plan that works with your body and schedule.

As you discover all that intermittent fasting can do for you, think of me as your guide—a mentor who understands what you're going through and is here to support you every step of the way. And, as with any health advice, please consult your physician, as I did on this journey.

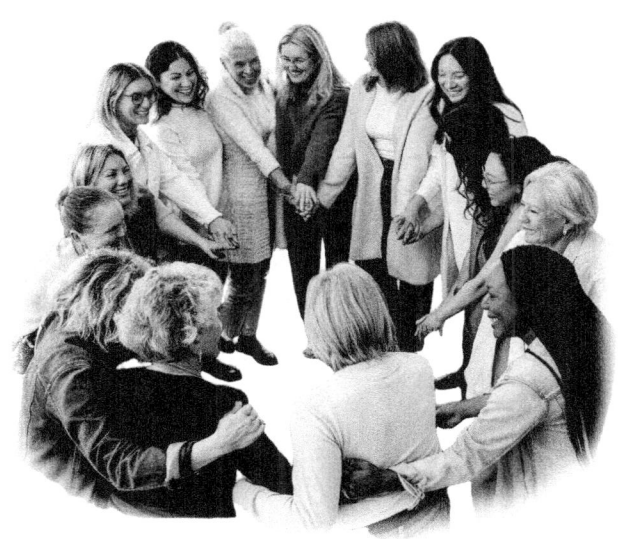

Remember to keep an open mind. Embrace this opportunity to make changes that will lead to a healthier, more energetic you. You have the power to transform your health and well-being. Let's take this journey together with hope, determination, and a sense of community.

1

INTERMITTENT FASTING AND HORMONAL HEALTH

"Take care of your body. It's the only place you have to live." — Jim Rohn

Have you ever found yourself halfway through the day, exhausted and wondering where all your energy went? I felt that way often, especially after turning forty. My body seemed to have its own agenda, which didn't quite align with my plans or energy needs. Around this time, I discovered intermittent fasting, which promised weight loss and offered a way to support my changing hormones and energy levels.

As we dive into this chapter, we'll explore how intermittent fasting can become a supportive tool in navigating the unique hormonal landscape of women over forty. You'll learn about the science behind fasting, how it differs from dieting, and why it might be the missing puzzle piece in your wellness journey.

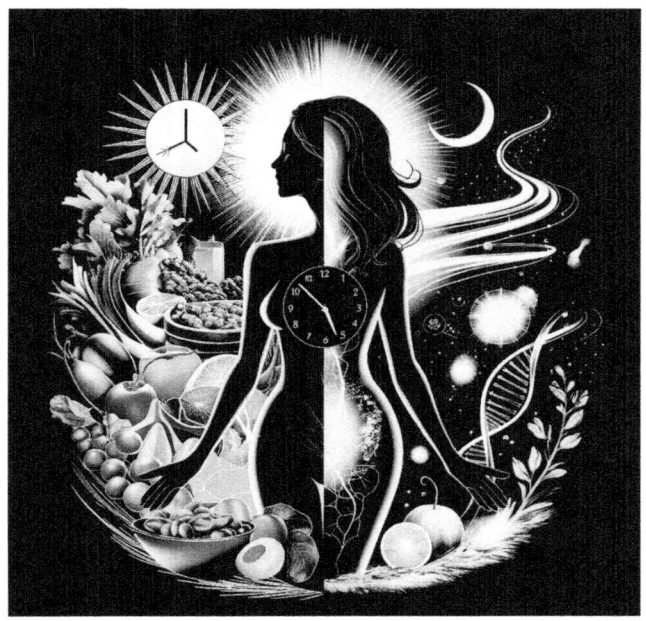

THE SCIENCE OF INTERMITTENT FASTING

Intermittent fasting, at its core, is about timing. It's not so much about what you eat but when you eat. You can eat whatever you want, but only during a specific time period. Although there are no strict guidelines for what you eat, you will have better results with a healthy, well-balanced diet.

This simple shift of alternating cycles of fasting and eating can lead to profound changes in how your body functions. One of the most fascinating aspects is cellular autophagy. A good analogy is thinking of your body as a house. Over time, clutter builds up. Autophagy is the natural process of decluttering. Your body cleans out damaged cells, making way for newer, healthier ones. This cellular spring cleaning renews your cells and supports your overall health. We'll talk more about autophagy in Chapter 6.

Another critical aspect of fasting is how it regulates hormones. Intermittent fasting helps balance insulin, which is essential for preventing insulin resistance, a common issue as we age. Lower insulin levels mean your body burns fat more efficiently, a process known as the metabolic switch. Instead of relying solely on glucose, your body uses stored fat for energy, which can help you lose weight and have more energy. Fasting can also enhance growth hormone production, which helps you maintain muscle and feel more resilient.

Fasting's holistic approach to health sets it apart from traditional dieting. Fasting doesn't just promise a thinner waistline. It offers a path to a healthier, more active life. Unlike diets that often feel restrictive and temporary, fasting aligns with your natural rhythms. This alignment can reduce inflammation, which is a critical factor in many age-related diseases.

Fasting has unique impacts on women, especially those over forty. Hormonal fluctuations during the menstrual cycle can affect how fasting works for you. During the follicular phase, when you feel more energetic, fasting might feel easier. The luteal phase, which can bring about PMS symptoms, might require a gentler approach. Understanding your cycle allows you to tailor fasting to your body's needs and enhance its effectiveness.

There are several fasting methods to choose from:

- The **16:8 method** is popular for its simplicity: You fast for sixteen hours and eat within an eight-hour window. This method easily fits into a typical day, allowing for late dinners or early breakfasts.
- The **5:2 method** involves eating normally for five days and reducing calorie intake on two nonconsecutive days.
- The **12:12 method** is perfect for beginners. You fast for twelve hours and eat with a twelve-hour window. The most important part is to not eat a late-night snack.
- The **14:10 method** is a nice intermediate step toward the 16:8 method or if fasting for sixteen hours doesn't work for you.

All methods offer flexibility, letting you find what works best for your lifestyle and body.

Your Fasting Starter Kit: If you're new to fasting, here's a simple checklist to help you get started:

- **Get a health screening:** A comprehensive health assessment is crucial. Your healthcare provider can help you evaluate key markers like hormone levels, thyroid function, insulin sensitivity, and overall metabolic health. This initial screening ensures that fasting is a safe and appropriate strategy for your individual health profile.
- **Set realistic expectations**: Intermittent fasting is not a quick fix. It's a lifestyle approach that requires patience and self-compassion. Understanding that progress is nonlinear and staying motivated through natural fluctuations in weight and energy is essential. Realistic expectations mean celebrating small victories, recognizing your body's unique journey, and focusing on overall wellness rather than just numerical changes.
- **Prepare mentally and focus on mindset shifts:** Beyond a physical adaptation, intermittent fasting requires a profound transformation in how you view nutrition, hunger, and self-care. Developing a compassionate, curious mindset allows you to approach this lifestyle change as an experiment in wellness, free from traditional dieting's shame and restrictions. Cultivating mental resilience means understanding that some days will be easier than others and that each experience is an opportunity for learning and growth.
- **Choose your method:** Decide between 16:8, 5:2, 12:12, or 14:10. Think about your schedule and what feels most manageable. Start with the 12:12 or 14:10 method and see how you feel before stepping up to the 16:8. When I

started, I started with the 14:10 and stuck with this method for a few weeks. Once my body got used to fasting, I moved to the 16:8 method.

- **16:8 method**
  - **What it is:** Fast for sixteen hours and eat during an eight-hour window.
  - **Typical schedule:** Skip breakfast, eat from noon to eight p.m., and fast until the next day, or eat late breakfast at ten a.m. and finish dinner by six p.m.
  - **Who it's suitable for:** Those looking for a simple, sustainable plan.
  - **Benefits:** Helps control calorie intake, supports weight loss, and aligns with natural eating patterns.
- **5:2 method**
  - **What it is:** Eat normally five days a week and consume only 500 to 600 calories on two nonconsecutive days.
  - **Typical schedule:** Eat normally on Monday, Wednesday, Friday, Saturday, and Sunday and restrict calories on Tuesday and Thursday.
  - **Who it's suitable for:** People who prefer flexibility and don't want to fast daily.
  - **Benefits:** Encourages calorie reduction without daily restrictions and supports fat loss.
- **12:12 method**
  - **What it is:** Fast for twelve hours and eat during a twelve-hour window.
  - **Typical schedule:** Eat your breakfast at eight a.m. and finish dinner by eight p.m.
  - **Who it's suitable for:** People who are starting intermittent fasting and want their bodies to adjust more easily.

- - **Benefits:** Helps control calorie intake and supports weight loss.
  - **14:10 method**
    - **What it is:** Fast for fourteen hours and eat during a ten-hour window.
    - **Typical schedule:** Eat a late breakfast at ten a.m. and finish dinner by eight p.m.
    - **Who it's suitable for:** Beginners and people who want a slightly longer eating window.
    - **Benefits:** Helps control calorie intake, supports weight loss, and aligns with natural eating patterns.
- **Plan your meals:** When you're in your eating window, focus on nutrient-dense foods. This doesn't mean you have to stay on a strict diet. However, planning meals is crucial because it helps you get the necessary nutrients, maintain energy levels, and make the most of your eating windows.
- **Exercise timing:** Many find success with working out toward the end of their fasting window or during the early hours of their eating window, which can maximize fat burning and muscle preservation. This approach allows you to leverage your body's metabolic state while ensuring that you have enough energy and nutrients for recovery and maintenance.
- **Strength training:** This becomes increasingly critical for women over forty, and intermittent fasting can be an excellent complement to preserving and developing muscle. Focusing on resistance training helps counteract age-related muscle loss, supports bone density, and boosts your metabolism more effectively than cardio alone. Pay special attention to protein intake during your eating windows and consider doing your most intense weight training sessions shortly after breaking your fast.

- **Energy management:** Understanding and managing your energy levels is important when integrating intermittent fasting with exercise. Your body may require a more nuanced approach to workout intensity, along with a focus on quality over quantity. You'll also want to allow for more rest and recovery time. Listening to your body, staying hydrated, and being willing to modify your exercise routine based on energy levels and hormonal fluctuations are essential for a long-term fitness plan.
- **Recovery and rest strategies:** Recovery becomes increasingly important as we age, making rest an integral part of your fitness and fasting strategy. Implement active recovery techniques like gentle stretching, foam rolling, and low-intensity movement on days when high-intensity workouts aren't possible.
- **Listen to your body:** Pay attention to how fasting feels and adjust as needed, especially around your menstrual cycle. While some discomfort is normal when first adapting, severe headaches, dizziness, or weakness indicate that you should break your fast. Pay attention to signs of dehydration, extreme fatigue, or difficulty concentrating. If you notice persistent negative symptoms, consider adjusting your fasting window or consulting a healthcare provider to find a more sustainable approach that works for your individual needs.
- **Stay hydrated:** Drink plenty of water during fasting periods to support cellular processes. This can't be emphasized enough. Hydration will also give you a feeling of fullness, which will be super helpful during fasting.
- **Track your progress:** Use a journal or app to track progress beyond the scale. Weight is just one of many indicators of health, and for women over forty, holistic

metrics are far more meaningful. Consider tracking energy levels, sleep quality, mood stability, muscle tone, clothing fit, and biomarkers, such as inflammation levels and insulin sensitivity. By expanding your definition of progress, you'll gain a more comprehensive understanding of how intermittent fasting is positively transforming your health.

These steps can set a solid foundation for incorporating intermittent fasting into your life. As you progress, remember that this is about finding balance and harmony with your body, not imposing restrictions.

Some practical tips that helped me early on in my journey were:

- **Plan for break-fast meals:** Include easily digestible, nutrient-dense foods to break your fast gently.
- **Batch cook:** Prepare meals in advance to save time and reduce effort.
- **Hydrate:** Plan fluids like water, herbal tea, or electrolytes during fasting hours to stay hydrated.
- **Snack strategically:** If your window allows, plan light snacks to prevent hunger spikes.

TAILORING FASTING TO FEMALE PHYSIOLOGY

When it comes to intermittent fasting, one size definitely does not fit all, especially for women navigating the complexities of their forties and beyond. Our bodies are like finely tuned instruments, each with its own melody and rhythm. It's important to tailor your approach to suit your unique hormonal profile and lifestyle so you can make fasting work for you.

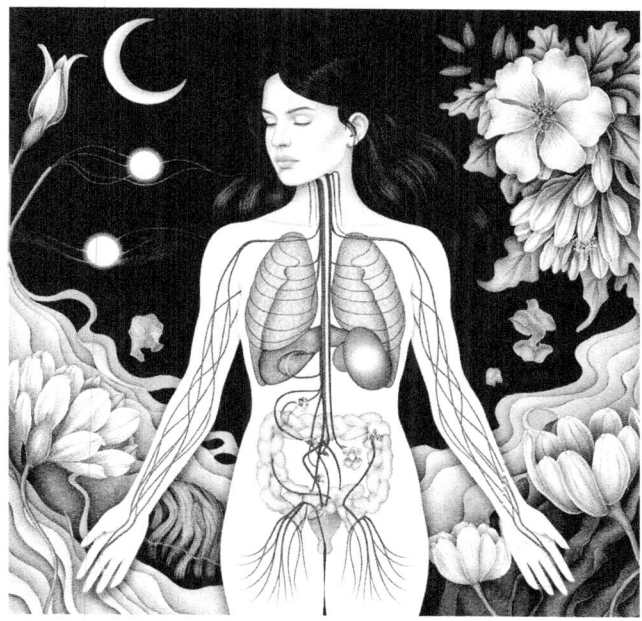

Start by assessing your needs. Consider keeping a journal to track symptoms, energy levels, and mood fluctuations. This self-evaluation can offer insights into how your menstrual cycle, stress, and daily routines interact with your fasting. By understanding your body's signals, you can modify your fasting plan to better support your well-being.

If you're still having menstrual cycles, you can adjust fasting to accommodate the natural ebb and flow of hormonal changes. During the luteal phase—the days leading up to menstruation—you might notice an increase in appetite or mood swings. To counter these effects, consider increasing your caloric intake slightly. Focus on nutrient-rich foods that satisfy cravings without derailing your fasting goals. By being mindful of these cyclical changes, you can keep your fasting practice consistent while honoring your body's needs.

Postmenopausal women have their own set of considerations. With the absence of menstrual cycles, the focus shifts slightly. Bone health becomes a top priority, given the reduced estrogen levels that can affect bone density. It's crucial to get adequate calcium and vitamin D. If you're postmenopausal, consider making leafy greens, fortified plant milks, and fatty fish staples in your diet. These foods support bone health and complement fasting by providing essential nutrients. Tailoring your fasting routine to your needs can help you stay strong and resilient.

Safety is a cornerstone of any fasting practice. Listen to your body and recognize any signs of nutrient deficiency or fatigue. Regularly assess your energy levels, skin health, and overall well-being. If you notice persistent fatigue, hair loss, or other concerning symptoms, it may be time to adjust your fasting plan or seek professional advice. Remember, fasting should feel sustainable and supportive, not like a strain on your health.

PERSONAL ASSESSMENT TOOL

To help you customize your fasting plan, here's a simple self-assessment tool:

- **Symptom tracker:** Note any changes in mood, energy, or physical symptoms throughout the month.
- **Lifestyle audit:** Review your daily schedule, stressors, and sleep patterns.
- **Nutrient checklist:** Consume foods rich in vitamins and minerals, particularly those that support bone and hormonal health.
- **Adjustment notes:** Record any fasting modifications and their effects on your well-being.

By regularly using this tool, you can make informed adjustments to your fasting routine so that it remains aligned with your health goals and life stage.

HORMONAL SHIFTS: NAVIGATING PERIMENOPAUSE, MENOPAUSE, AND BEYOND

As you move through your forties and beyond, your body embarks on a new phase. It's a time marked by hormonal shifts that can feel like a roller-coaster ride. During perimenopause—the transition leading up to menopause—estrogen levels begin to fluctuate. This hormone plays a crucial role in regulating mood and body weight. As it declines, you might notice weight shifting to different areas of your body. It often settles around the midsection. And if you are like me, you'll likely have mood swings that feel like they come out of nowhere. It's not just estrogen that causes changes. Progesterone, another critical hormone, also fluctuates. For me, this caused sleepless nights and more anxiety.

These hormonal shifts can feel overwhelming, but there's a silver lining. Intermittent fasting can offer stability amid the chaos. Giving your body regular breaks from eating gives your hormonal system a chance to recalibrate. For instance, many women who fast report fewer hot flashes. This is because fasting can help balance hormone levels and create a more stable internal environment. Moreover, it can help smooth out mood swings, leaving you feeling more in control and less at the mercy of hormonal tides.

Now let's talk about how to tailor fasting to support these changes. Timing is everything. Consider aligning your fasting windows with your symptom patterns. If hot flashes flare up at night, an earlier eating window might help. Similarly, if anxiety peaks in the afternoon, break your fast with calming, nutrient-rich meals to get the support you need. The flexibility of intermittent fasting allows you to adjust your habits to your daily realities, which helps you feel the best you can through these hormonal changes.

Sarah's Story: Real-life experiences can be incredibly powerful in showing us how fasting can help. Take Sarah, a woman who shared her story with me. In her late forties,

Sarah struggled with intense mood swings and hot flashes. She tried supplements and prescription medication but with little success. After incorporating intermittent fasting, she noticed a remarkable difference. She used the self-assessment tool to document her symptoms and stressors and then adjusted her eating window, which made her feel calmer and more in control. Her story is one of many that illustrate how fasting can be a practical tool in navigating this life stage.

Experts in the field also speak to the benefits of fasting. Dr. Jolene Brighten, a leading expert in women's health, discusses the benefits of intermittent fasting during menopause, noting that it can aid in weight control, balance hormones by improving insulin levels, and reduce menopausal symptoms like hot flashes. Such insights from the medical community provide a credible backdrop to personal testimonials, reinforcing the potential of fasting as a supportive practice during perimenopause and menopause.

As you explore fasting, remember that it's a personal journey. What works for one woman might not work for another, and that's perfectly okay. The key lies in listening to your body and making adjustments that honor your unique needs. Consider keeping a symptom journal, noting how you feel during different fasting windows. This can help you identify patterns and make informed decisions about your fasting practice. Ultimately, the goal is to find a rhythm that supports your hormonal health and lifestyle, allowing you to embrace this new phase with confidence.

ADDRESSING MENOPAUSE BELLY WITH FASTING

Menopause belly. It's a term many of us become all too familiar with as we navigate our forties and beyond. You're not alone if you've noticed a shift in your waistline, with fat accumulating more stubbornly around the abdomen. This isn't just about aesthetics. Deeper hormonal and metabolic reasons are at play.

As estrogen levels decline, the body tends to store more fat centrally. This shift is linked to increased insulin resistance. Insulin, a hormone that helps your cells use glucose for energy, can become less effective, prompting your body to store more fat, especially around the belly.

But there's hope in understanding these mechanisms. Intermittent fasting can be a powerful tool in addressing these changes. By providing regular breaks from food, fasting helps improve insulin sensitivity, allowing your body to manage glucose more effectively. This improved sensitivity means you're less inclined to store excess fat, particularly around the abdomen. Fasting taps into your fat reserves and targets visceral fat—the type that wraps around your organs and poses significant health risks—more effectively than traditional dieting.

Pairing fasting with the right exercises can enhance these effects. Strength training, in particular, is a fantastic complement to fasting. It boosts your metabolism and helps you build lean muscle mass. And that naturally burns more calories when you're at rest. Consider incorporating squats, lunges, and deadlifts into your routine. These movements engage multiple muscle groups, making them efficient and effective. Aim for two to three weekly strength training sessions, allowing your muscles time to recover and grow stronger. This combination of fasting and strength training can be transformative, helping you tackle menopause belly from multiple angles.

Dietary adjustments also play a crucial role. While fasting focuses on when you eat, what you eat during your eating windows matters significantly. Incorporate anti-inflammatory foods to support both fasting and fat loss:

- **Turmeric**, renowned for its anti-inflammatory properties, can be an excellent addition to your diet. Try adding it to smoothies or use it to season soups and stews.

- **Leafy greens**—rich in vitamins and antioxidants—should also feature prominently in your meals. Think kale, spinach, and Swiss chard. These powerhouses nourish your body and support hormonal balance.
- Include a variety of **colorful vegetables, lean proteins (chicken breasts, egg whites, and fish), and healthy fats (avocados and nuts)**, to create balanced, satisfying meals that align with your fasting goals.

My typical day might start with a nourishing smoothie packed with greens and a dash of turmeric, followed by a hearty salad with grilled chicken for lunch. Dinner may be a warm, comforting stew loaded with vegetables and lean protein.

This type of approach gives you the necessary nutrients while supporting fat loss and overall health. Remember, consistency is key. Changes won't happen overnight, but with dedication and persistence, you'll begin to see and feel the difference.

By understanding the causes of menopause belly and taking a targeted approach through fasting, exercise, and diet, you can reclaim your waistline and boost your overall health.

EMPOWERING WOMEN THROUGH HORMONAL HARMONY

Intermittent fasting is more than a tool for weight management. It's a means of empowerment, particularly for women over forty. As you navigate the complexities of hormonal changes, fasting offers a way to take back control over your health.

In a world where many factors may seem beyond your grasp, fasting is something you can choose and adapt to your needs. It aligns with your body's natural rhythms, providing a sense of autonomy and mastery over your well-being. By making informed choices about when and how you eat, you can influence your energy, mood, and long-term health outcomes. This empowerment comes not just from the physical changes you might see but from the psychological strength you gain in knowing you're actively participating in your health journey.

A key component of this empowerment is community support. I have found that engaging with others who share similar goals and challenges can be incredibly motivating. Whether you find one through online forums, local meetups, or even book clubs centered around wellness, a community offers belonging and a shared experience. It's comforting to know that others are walking a similar path and facing the same ups and downs. Sharing stories, exchanging tips, and celebrating successes can make the difference between giving up and pressing on. This collective journey fosters resilience and provides a support network that uplifts and encourages each woman to continue striving for her goals.

Fasting also brings emotional and psychological benefits that are often overlooked. The structured eating patterns inherent in fasting can help reduce stress by eliminating the constant decision-making around food. Knowing when you'll have your next meal and having a plan can free up mental space and reduce anxiety. For me, this predictability has been incredibly soothing during my hormonal fluctuations, when uncertainty about how I'll feel from one moment to the next can be unsettling. Moreover, fasting encourages you to be self-aware and mindful. And that fosters a deeper connection with your body and how it responds to different stimuli.

Mindful eating becomes a natural extension of fasting. It allows you to savor your meals, appreciate the flavors and textures, and truly enjoy the act of eating. This mindfulness can enhance the benefits of fasting because it promotes better digestion and a more satisfying eating experience. It's about being present and intentional, and each meal becomes a moment of nourishment and pleasure rather than a rushed necessity. This shift in perspective can transform your relationship with food, making it less about restriction and more about nourishment and enjoyment.

To maximize the benefits of intermittent fasting, it's helpful to integrate it with other wellness practices. Yoga and meditation are excellent complements to fasting, offering additional tools for managing stress and supporting overall health. Yoga can help keep your body flexible and strong, while meditation provides a space to quiet your mind and center yourself. Together, these practices create a holistic approach to wellness that addresses both physical and mental health. They encourage a balance that can be particularly beneficial during periods of hormonal change, providing stability and calm.

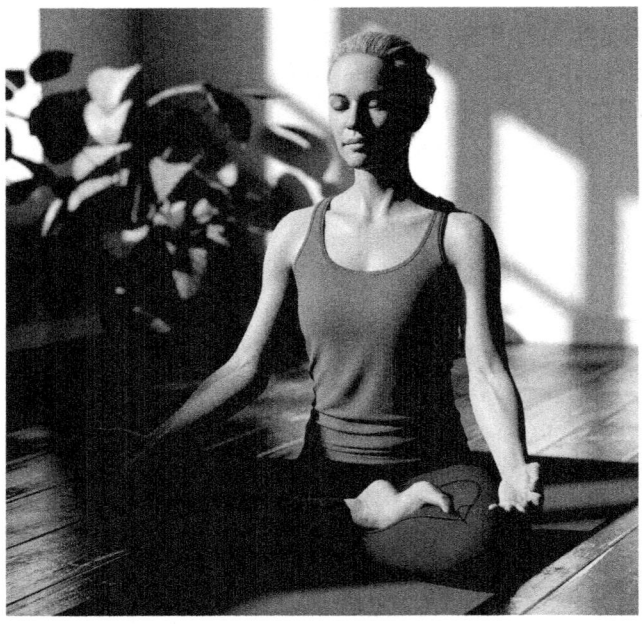

As you embrace fasting, you'll find it's not just about physical change. It's an invitation to explore what it means to feel empowered and capable. This holistic approach considers your body, mind, and spirit, integrating various aspects of your life into a cohesive whole. By taking control of your health in this way, you create a foundation for a healthier, more energetic, and more fulfilling life. With each small step, from choosing your fasting windows to engaging with supportive communities, you can build a life that reflects your strengths and aspirations. Here, you find harmony—not just with your hormones but with yourself.

OVERCOMING COMMON MISCONCEPTIONS ABOUT FASTING AND HORMONES

Starting intermittent fasting can feel confusing with all the myths floating around. One of the most pervasive misconceptions is the fear of muscle loss. Many women worry that by fasting, they might lose the very muscle mass they've worked hard to build. However, it's important to understand that our bodies are incredibly adaptive. During fasting, the body doesn't just haphazardly break down muscle for energy. Instead, it taps into fat stores while maintaining muscle integrity. This is mainly due to the role of protein synthesis, which continues even during fasting. Growth hormone levels rise during fasting, supporting muscle maintenance. The body is designed to preserve muscle mass despite limited food intake. It's a survival mechanism, ensuring that we don't lose essential muscle tissue during times of scarcity.

Another common myth is confusing fasting with starvation. Fasting, when done correctly, is a controlled practice with defined periods of eating and not eating. Starvation, on the other hand, is an extended lack of food that leads to severe nutrient deficiencies and health issues. Intermittent fasting doesn't deprive the body of necessary nutrients. In fact, it encourages a focus on nutritional adequacy. That's why it's crucial to consume a balanced diet rich in essential nutrients during eating windows. This gives your body what it needs to function optimally and supports everything from hormone production to immune function. It's about quality, not just quantity. Incorporating nutrient-dense foods—such as lean proteins (low-fat dairy, lentils, and turkey breasts), healthy fats, and a rainbow of fruits and vegetables—can make a significant difference.

Scientific studies bolster the benefits of fasting, especially concerning hormonal balance. For instance, research indicates that fasting may affect reproductive hormone levels in women by decreasing androgen markers, like testosterone, while increasing sex hormone-binding globulin levels. These changes can be particularly beneficial for women dealing with conditions like polycystic ovary syndrome.[1] Such findings underscore the potential of fasting as a tool for improving hormonal health.

Moreover, fasting has been shown to optimize insulin function, reducing the risk of type 2 diabetes—a significant concern as we age.[2] These insights are empowering and provide a scientific backbone to the anecdotal evidence many women share about their positive experiences with fasting.

Making informed decisions about fasting begins with knowledge. While the benefits of fasting can be profound, it's essential to consult with healthcare providers before starting any new regimen. They can offer personalized advice, ensuring that fasting aligns with your individual health needs and lifestyle. This step is particularly important if you have preexisting medical conditions or take medications. Your healthcare provider can help you tailor a fasting plan that supports your health goals without compromising safety.

To support your journey, consider creating a list of questions to discuss with your healthcare provider. This could include how to integrate fasting with current health conditions, how fasting might interact with medications, or even how to monitor nutrient intake effectively. Here's a simple checklist to guide your conversation:

---

1. Sophia Cienfuegos, Sarah Corapi, Kelsey Gabel, Mark Ezpeleta, Faiza Kalam, Shuhao Lin, Vasiliki Pavlou, and Krista A. Varaday, "Effects of Intermittent Fasting on Reproductive Hormone Levels in Females and Males: A Review of Human Trials," April 22, 2022, the MPDI website, https://www.mdpi.com/2072-6643/14/11/2343.

2. Emily Borgundvaag, Jessica Mak, and Caroline K. Kramer, "Metabolic Impact of Intermittent Fasting in Patients With Type 2 Diabetes Mellitus: A Systematic Review and Meta-analysis of Interventional Studies," *The Journal of Clinical Endocrinology and Metabolism* 106 no. 3 (2021): 902-11.

CONSULTATION CHECKLIST

- **Discuss health history:** Share your medical history and any current medications.
- **Ask about nutrient intake:** Inquire about maintaining nutritional adequacy during fasting.
- **Explore fasting schedules:** Discuss which fasting methods might suit your lifestyle.
- **Monitor hormonal changes:** Talk about tracking any hormonal changes and their impacts.

Navigating the world of intermittent fasting with the correct information and guidance allows you to make empowering and informed choices that equip you to embrace fasting as a supportive tool in your wellness tool kit.

2

CYCLE-SPECIFIC FASTING

"Your body whispers before it screams." — Dr. Elizabeth Boham

Think about how it would feel to wake up each day with renewed energy, feeling in sync with your body rather than at odds with it. For many of us, the menstrual cycle can feel like a roller coaster, with each phase bringing its own challenges and surprises. Over time, I realized that instead of resisting these changes, it might be more effective to align my lifestyle with them. This led me to the concept of cycle-specific fasting. This approach respects the body's natural rhythms and enhances the benefits of intermittent fasting by aligning it with the menstrual cycle.

During the follicular phase, which kicks off right after menstruation and lasts about nine days, estrogen and progesterone rise, resulting in higher energy levels and a more positive mood (this is according to Mayo Clinic and WebMD). You might feel more adventurous and open to trying new things. Fasting during this phase can be particularly effective, as your body is energetic and more adaptable to changes in eating patterns. Many women find they can easily extend their fasting windows, making it a great time to experiment with fasting durations like the 16:8 method, in which you eat during an eight-hour window and fast for sixteen. You might feel more inclined to engage in intense workouts or tackle challenging projects, as your body is naturally primed for activity and endurance.

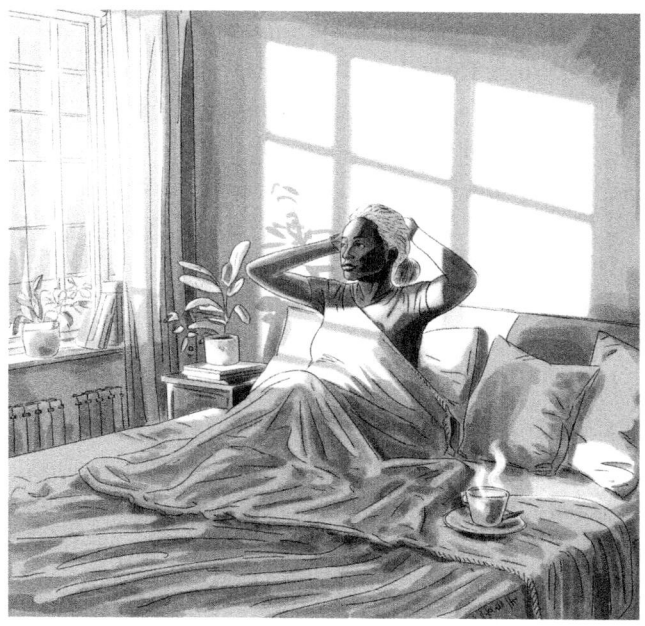

As you transition into the luteal phase, the dynamic changes. This phase, which lasts about ten days, is marked by high, then decreasing, hormone levels. You might feel anxiety and the notorious PMS symptoms. Your calorie demand can increase, and cravings might seem overwhelming. This is where a gentler approach to fasting can be beneficial. Consider shortening your fasting window to something like the 14:10 method. It allows you to maintain the benefits of fasting while accommodating your heightened need for nourishment and comfort. Focus on foods rich in healthy fats (avocados, nuts, olive oil, fatty fishes, and eggs) and slow-digesting carbohydrates (quinoa, sweet potatoes, steel-cut oats, fruits, vegetables, and legumes), which can help stabilize mood and energy levels.

Aligning your fasting practices with these hormonal fluctuations, a process known as cycle syncing, offers numerous benefits. Tailored fasting can help balance hormones, reduce the severity of PMS symptoms, and support overall well-being. Women who have embraced this approach often report that they feel more in tune with their bodies, have fewer mood swings, and enjoy more consistent energy levels throughout the month. It's about working with your body, not against it, and creating harmony between your lifestyle and biological rhythms.

In practice, a cycle-synced fasting routine might look like this:

- **Follicular phase:** You might start with a longer fasting window, perhaps from eight p.m. to noon the next day. This allows your body to capitalize on its natural energy boost.
- **Luteal phase:** You could adjust your eating window, perhaps from eight p.m. to ten a.m., to accommodate any increased hunger or cravings. The key is being flexible and listening to what your body needs at each stage.

Emily's Story: A good friend of mine named Emily struggled with severe PMS and energy crashes before she tried cycle syncing. After aligning her fasting and eating habits with her menstrual phases for a few months, she noticed dramatically fewer physical and emotional symptoms. By increasing her caloric intake slightly during the luteal phase and focusing on nutrient-dense foods, Emily maintained her fasting routine without the distress she used to feel. Her story shows how powerful and transformative cycle syncing can be.

CYCLE SYNCING REFLECTION

Consider taking a moment each week to reflect on aligning your fasting and menstrual cycle. Ask yourself:

- "How have my energy levels been this week?"
- "Did I notice any changes in cravings or mood?"
- "What adjustments can I make to better support my body in the coming days?"

Integrating these reflections into your routine allows you to fine-tune your fasting to suit your needs, fostering a deeper connection with your body and its natural rhythms.

FASTING STRATEGIES FOR WOMEN WITHOUT MENSTRUAL CYCLES

After menopause, the landscape of health changes considerably. The end of menstruation brings about a new phase that calls for a thoughtful approach to maintaining wellness. Fasting can be a powerful tool to help you manage these shifts.

Bone health is one key area. With the decline in estrogen, your bones may become more susceptible to thinning, increasing the risk of osteoporosis. A diet rich in calcium can help. Leafy greens, fortified plant-based milks, and almonds can support strong bones. Coupling this nutritional strategy with fasting can enhance your body's ability to utilize these nutrients effectively to support bone density and overall strength and resilience.

Flexibility is the cornerstone of fasting if you're postmenopausal. As your body no longer follows the cyclical patterns of menstruation, your fasting routine must adapt. The 16:8 method offers a balanced approach that can fit seamlessly into daily life. This method supports metabolic health without the pressure of strict time constraints. I have personally stayed on this method the longest but have shifted to 14:10 or 12:12 during periods of travel or when my schedule gets out of sync.

Alternate-day fasting (switching between fasting and eating every twenty-four hours) allows for a more relaxed schedule. And that's beneficial if you prefer flexibility in your eating patterns. It's about listening to your body and adjusting as needed. You might find that some days call for longer eating windows, and that's perfectly okay. The goal is to create a fasting practice that serves your current health needs and lifestyle.

While the absence of a menstrual cycle might seem like a loss of rhythm, it's actually an opportunity to embrace the universal advantages of fasting. These benefits go beyond menstruation to support weight management, cognitive clarity, and metabolic health.

Fasting helps improve insulin sensitivity, which is crucial for managing your weight and reducing your risk of type 2 diabetes. It's also good for your brain function, helping you have a clearer mind and better focus. These benefits are not tied to any one phase of life, making them accessible to all women of all ages.

The freedom that comes from this kind of fasting is profound. It's an approach that respects your body's signals, allowing you to engage with fasting on your own terms.

Health experts offer valuable insights into fasting for women without cycles. Dr. Jolene Brighten, a leading expert in women's health, suggests that intermittent fasting can aid in weight control and balance hormones by improving insulin levels, which supports better blood sugar control. She emphasizes the importance of choosing a fasting method that fits your lifestyle and gradually integrating it into daily routines while paying close attention to your body's response.[1]

According to Dr. Brighten, unwanted weight gain—often around the midsection or even obesity —often becomes a major concern during menopause, as metabolic rates slow down and fat distribution shifts, making weight management more challenging. However, fasting has been shown to help, including by lowering caloric intake and supporting hormonal balance.

---

1. Jolene Brighten, NMD, FABNE, "Intermittent Fasting for Menopause: What You Need to Know Before You Start," December 29, 2023, the Dr. Jolene Brighten website, https://drbrighten.com/intermittent-fasting-for-menopause/?utm_source=chatgpt.com.

Interactive Element: Personal Fasting Flexibility Plan
Consider creating a personalized fasting plan for your current lifestyle and health goals. Use the following prompts to guide you:

- **Identify your energy peaks:** When do you feel most energetic during the day? Tailor your eating window to these times.
- **Nutrient focus:** List three calcium-rich foods you enjoy and incorporate them into your meals.
- **Weekly reflection:** At the end of each week, take a few minutes to jot down what worked well and what might need adjusting in your fasting and eating schedule. How did your energy levels respond to different fasting windows?

I found that I had the most energy in the mornings. So, starting my fasting at noon or after worked well for me. After several weeks of engaging with these prompts, I developed a fasting strategy that aligns best with my body—a meal plan with foods that I enjoyed eating and that gave me the most energy throughout the day. Doing the same thing will help you make sure your practice remains effective and enjoyable.

ADJUSTING FASTING DURING PERIMENOPAUSE

Perimenopause can make you feel like your body is playing a game of hormonal hopscotch. Just as you think you've found your footing, something shifts. Progesterone, a key player in this phase, fluctuates unpredictably. This hormone, which once provided a calming effect, now ebbs and flows, influencing your mood and appetite in unexpected ways. One moment, you might feel on top of the world, and the next, you're reaching for comfort foods. These changes can make fasting seem daunting, but by understanding how these hormones impact your body, you can adjust your fasting to better suit your needs.

Time-restricted eating is a valuable strategy during perimenopause. It involves eating all your meals in a specific window of time each day, such as ten hours, which can help manage hormonal energy fluctuations. By structuring your eating periods, you provide your body with a consistent routine. And this can be particularly comforting during unpredictable hormonal changes. You can choose windows that align with your energy levels, making it easier to manage day-to-day tasks and commitments without feeling drained. You might find it best to start your eating window later in the morning and close it earlier in the evening, as it allows for a longer fasting period overnight and gives your body time to reset.

Perimenopause can also bring a host of symptoms, notably hot flashes. These sudden surges of heat can be disruptive, affecting everything from sleep to work. Interestingly, intermittent fasting may offer some relief.

By regulating metabolic processes, fasting can help stabilize your body temperature and reduce the frequency and intensity of hot flashes. Fasting helps balance insulin and glucose levels, which in turn may contribute to a more stable internal thermostat. Tailoring your fasting schedule to these symptoms can make a significant difference. For instance, if hot flashes tend to occur at night, you might consider ending your eating window earlier in the evening, allowing your body to focus on resting rather than digesting. This strategy has helped me tremendously. Journaling identified that as I shifted to eating earlier—six p.m. vs. seven-thirty p.m.—I experienced a drastic reduction in hot flashes in the middle of the night.

Of course, fasting during perimenopause isn't without its challenges. Hydration becomes particularly important, as it helps counteract the dehydration of hot flashes and supports overall health during fasting. Drink plenty of water and consider herbal teas, like chamomile or peppermint, which can soothe your digestive system and provide a moment of calm.

Nutrition also plays a critical role. Focus on nutrient-dense foods that pack a punch, such as leafy greens, nuts, seeds, and lean proteins. They can help replenish your nutrients, keeping energy levels steady and mood swings at bay.

Common hurdles during perimenopause can include cravings and emotional eating driven by hormonal turbulence. When you find yourself reaching for that extra snack, pause and ask yourself if it's from hunger or habit. Mindful eating practices can be a great ally here, helping you make conscious choices about what and when you eat. Consider keeping a journal to track your meals and symptoms, noting how different foods and fasting windows affect your mood and energy. This self-awareness can help you make healthy adjustments.

COPING STRATEGIES CHECKLIST

- **Hydration:** Keep a water bottle handy and sip throughout the day. Herbal teas are a great option for variety.
- **Nutrient-dense foods:** Prioritize leafy greens, lean proteins, and healthy fats (fatty fish, eggs, dark chocolate, nut butter, and cheese).
- **Mindful eating:** Slow down during meals, savor each bite, and listen to your body's hunger cues.
- **Symptom tracking:** Use a journal to record eating habits, symptoms, and mood changes.

By incorporating these strategies, you can navigate perimenopause with greater ease, allowing fasting to become a supportive element in your routine.

MENOPAUSE-SPECIFIC FASTING PROTOCOLS

Many women find themselves seeking relief from the constant hot flashes and night sweats of menopause, and intermittent fasting offers a promising avenue. It can help you manage the symptoms—particularly those pesky hot flashes.

When you fast, your body undergoes metabolic regulation that can stabilize insulin and glucose levels. This stabilization helps reduce the frequency and intensity of hot flashes. Giving your body a break from constant digestion allows it to focus on balancing hormones. This break provides a more stable internal environment.

If you're in menopause, the 12:12 fasting schedule can be particularly beneficial. It involves fasting for twelve hours and eating within the next twelve-hour period. It's a gentle introduction to fasting that helps maintain energy levels while offering the metabolic benefits needed to manage menopausal symptoms. You can easily fit this schedule into a typical day, allowing for flexibility in meal timing. And that's essential when dealing with fluctuating energy levels. Women have found that this method offers a sustainable way to incorporate fasting into daily life without feeling deprived or overwhelmed.

Diet plays a significant role in supporting fasting during menopause. Phytoestrogen-rich foods can offer additional benefits. Flaxseeds, soybeans, and lentils contain natural compounds that mimic estrogen in the body. They can help balance hormones naturally, offering relief from some of the more challenging menopause symptoms.

A typical day might include:

- **Breakfast:** Smoothie with flaxseeds
- **Lunch:** Lentil soup
- **Dinner:** Tofu stir-fry

These meals support hormonal health and give you the nutrients you need to keep energy levels stable throughout the day.

Lisa's Story: My friend Lisa had been struggling with severe hot flashes and fatigue. She decided to try intermittent fasting, starting with the 12:12 method. Within a few weeks, she noticed a significant reduction in her symptoms. The hot flashes that once disrupted her sleep and daily activities became less frequent and intense. She also found that after she incorporated flaxseeds into her meals, she felt more balanced and energized.

Menopause is a time of significant transition, and it's important to approach fasting with patience and kindness toward yourself. Consider starting with the 12:12 schedule, then gradually explore other fasting methods as you become more comfortable. Remember, your body is adapting to a new phase, and it's okay to take things one step at a time. Listen to how your body responds and make adjustments as needed. If twelve hours feels manageable, you might experiment with extending the fasting window slightly. The key is to find a routine that fits seamlessly into your lifestyle and supports your health without adding stress.

POSTMENOPAUSE: MAINTAINING BALANCE WITH FASTING

Entering the postmenopausal phase is like stepping into a new chapter that allows for reflection and renewal. The body has settled into a new rhythm, and fasting can play a significant role in maintaining balance.

The 16:8 method is one effective and sustainable fasting strategy for postmenopausal women. Since it involves fasting for sixteen hours daily, followed by an eight-hour eating window, it's straightforward and aligns well with the body's natural metabolic processes.

It also offers consistent benefits, like improved insulin sensitivity and weight management. Many women find this method fits seamlessly into their routines and allows them to enjoy meals during the day while giving the body a substantial overnight fast to reset and repair.

Fasting does more than help you manage symptoms. It encourages a holistic approach to health, emphasizing overall wellness. It supports your body's natural detoxification processes, boosts metabolic efficiency, and can even enhance cognitive function. This holistic focus is crucial after menopause, when maintaining vigor and mental clarity becomes increasingly important. Women often report feeling more alert and focused, and they experience less of the brain fog that can sometimes accompany hormonal shifts. Engaging in regular fasting practices can create balance, not just physically but mentally, contributing to a more harmonious lifestyle.

Emotional well-being is another critical aspect to consider. As hormonal fluctuations settle, you might still experience emotional changes that require attention and care. Incorporating mindfulness into your fasting routine can provide emotional stability. Mindfulness encourages you to be present, helping you manage stress and reduce anxiety. You can integrate meditation or simple deep-breathing exercises into your daily routine, especially during fasting periods. They offer calm and enhance the benefits of fasting by promoting a centered and balanced state of mind. Taking a few moments each day for mindfulness can transform your fasting experience into a time of reflection and self-care.

Community support can be invaluable. Engaging with others on a similar path provides encouragement and belonging. Online forums dedicated to fasting and wellness are excellent places to start. These platforms allow you to connect with other women, share experiences, and exchange advice. Finding a community that understands your unique challenges can make all the difference. It's reassuring to know that others are navigating similar waters, and their insights can offer practical solutions and motivation. Whether you discuss fasting techniques or simply share personal stories, these connections can strengthen your resolve and enhance your fasting journey.

Incorporating fasting into your postmenopausal life doesn't have to be overwhelming. It's about finding a rhythm that works for you—one that respects your body's needs and supports your overall health goals.

NAVIGATING HORMONAL FLUCTUATIONS WITH FLEXIBLE FASTING

Navigating the ever-shifting landscape of hormonal changes can feel like a dance with an unpredictable partner. Flexibility is key. Intermittent fasting, when approached with adaptability, becomes a valuable ally. Instead of rigid schedules, consider intuitive fasting, in which you listen to your body's cues and adjust your eating windows accordingly. Your body knows what it needs, but you sometimes have to pay a little extra attention to decode its signals. One day, you may find that a longer fast feels natural, while another day, a shorter eating window fits better. This flexibility can reduce stress and help you make fasting a long-term part of your lifestyle.

Regular self-assessment becomes a crucial component of your fasting practice. By monitoring symptoms, you gain insights into how fasting affects your body and mind. Journals and apps can be valuable tools in this process. They help you track patterns, like energy levels, mood changes, and physical symptoms. This data empowers you to decide when to adjust your fasting windows. For instance, if you notice a dip in energy one week, it might signal you to tweak your fasting schedule or incorporate more nutrient-dense foods. Tracking can foster a deeper connection with your body, encouraging mindfulness and self-awareness.

Personalization is at the heart of a successful fasting routine. What works for one person might not work for another, and that's perfectly okay. Fasting logs are a great way to track your progress and customize your approach. These logs can include your fasting hours, meals, and changes in symptoms or energy. Over time, you'll see patterns that offer valuable insights into what adjustments might be beneficial. You may find that certain foods enhance your energy levels or that one fasting window aligns better with your natural rhythms. This personalization transforms fasting from a generic practice into a tailored strategy that meets your unique needs.

As with any lifestyle change, fasting comes with challenges. Plateaus, for instance, are common and can be frustrating. Your progress might stall despite your best efforts. When this happens, it's important to remember that plateaus are a natural part of the process. They often signal that it's time to reassess and adjust. Consider experimenting with your fasting windows—perhaps fasting every other day or incorporating a longer fast once a week. These changes can jump-start your progress, helping you overcome the plateau and continue moving forward. It's about finding a balance that works for you and supports your health goals without feeling restrictive.

The flexibility inherent in this approach encourages empowerment. By listening to your body and making adjustments as needed, you take control of your health. This adaptability enhances fasting's effectiveness and makes it a sustainable part of your life. As you navigate your hormonal fluctuations, let flexibility be your guide. Embrace the changes, trust your instincts, and allow your fasting practice to evolve with you.

As we wrap up our exploration of cycle-specific fasting, remember that your body is unique. Its needs will change over time. Embrace the journey and let fasting be a tool that supports you through these transitions.

3
NUTRITIONAL FOUNDATIONS FOR SUCCESSFUL FASTING

"Let food be thy medicine and medicine be thy food." — *Hippocrates*

I remember standing in the grocery aisle, staring at the colorful array of products and feeling overwhelmed by the sheer variety, unsure which foods would best nourish my body. It's no secret that as women over forty, our nutritional needs have shifted.

You require a diet that supports your body's natural rhythms and complements your fasting practices. In this chapter, we'll explore how to build a nutrient-dense plate that aligns with your health goals and enhances your fasting experience.

At the heart of a successful fasting regimen lies a foundation of essential micronutrients. These tiny powerhouses play a critical role in maintaining health, especially during fasting:

- **Iron** is essential for moving oxygen and making hormones, so it's crucial for energy. Lean meats, beans, and spinach are excellent sources, and pairing them with foods rich in vitamin C can enhance absorption.

- **Calcium** is essential for bone health, particularly as we age. Incorporating dairy, fortified plant milks, and leafy greens can ensure that you're meeting your calcium needs.
- **Omega-3 fatty acids**, found in fatty fish and flaxseeds, help reduce inflammation and support heart health.

Creating a balanced plate means embracing diverse food groups to ensure that you get the right mix of proteins, fats, and carbohydrates:

- **Proteins** from chicken, tofu, and legumes help maintain muscle mass and support metabolism.
- **Healthy fats**, such as those in avocados and nuts, provide a sense of fullness and are essential for hormone production.
- **Carbohydrates**, particularly from whole grains and colorful vegetables, offer energy and are rich in antioxidants, which combat oxidative stress. Some leafy greens (like Swiss chard and spinach) are particularly beneficial, offering a wealth of vitamins and minerals that support overall health.

By including a variety of these foods, you can create a diet that nourishes your body and aligns with your fasting goals.

Fiber is an unsung hero in the world of nutrition, playing a key role in both feeling full and digestion. Foods rich in fiber, like whole grains and legumes, help keep you feeling full longer, reducing the temptation to snack outside your eating window. They also support digestive health, promote regularity, and help maintain a healthy weight. Incorporating fiber-rich foods into your meals can help you stay satisfied and energized, making it easier to stick to your fasting plan. Consider starting your day with oatmeal topped with berries or enjoying a hearty lentil stew for lunch to boost your fiber intake.

FOOD LIST INTERMITTENT FASTING

MEATS
- Bacon
- Beef
- Chicken
- Eggs
- Pork
- Sausage
- Turkey

SEAFOOD
- Clams
- Cod
- Crab
- Tilapia
- Tuna
- Salmon
- Sardines
- Scallops
- Shrimp
- Trout

WHOLE GRAINS
- Ancient Grains
- Brown Rice
- Corn
- Oats
- Popcorn
- Quinoa
- Rice
- Sweet Potatoes
- Whole Grain Pasta

FRUITS
- Apples
- Apricots
- Avocado
- Bananas
- Blackberries
- Blueberries
- Cherries
- Grapefruit
- Kiwi
- Lemons
- Lime
- Oranges
- Peaches
- Pears
- Plums
- Raspberries
- Strawberries
- Watermelon

NUTS & SEEDS
- Almonds
- Cashews
- Chia Seeds
- Flax Seeds
- Hemp Seeds
- Macadamia
- Pecans
- Pine Nuts
- Pistachios
- Walnuts

VEGETABLES
- Acorn Squash
- Asparagus
- Beets
- Bell Peppers
- Bok Choy
- Broccoli
- Brussels Sprouts
- Butternut Squash
- Cabbage
- Carrots
- Cauliflower
- Cucumbers
- Eggplant
- Garlic
- Green Beans
- Kale
- Lettuce
- Onions
- Spaghetti Squash
- Spinach
- Summer Squash
- Zucchini

FATS & OILS
- Avocado Oil
- Coconut Oil
- Cooking Oil
- Olive Oil
- Sesame Oil
- Vegetable Oil

FROZEN
- Fruits (unsweetened)
- Meat
- Stir-Fry Veggie Mixes
- Seafood
- Vegetables

DAIRY & MILK
- Butter
- Cream
- Dairy Milk
- Cheese
- Coconut Milk
- Ghee
- Half & Half
- Non-Dairy Milk

SAUCES & MORE
- BBQ
- Buffalo Sauce
- Coconut Aminos
- Coffee
- Hot Sauce
- Ketchup
- Mayonnaise
- Mustard
- Peanut Butter
- Salad Dressing
- Soy Sauce
- Tea
- Vinegar

VISUAL GUIDE: BUILDING A NUTRIENT-DENSE PLATE

Creating a balanced meal doesn't have to be complicated. Use the following visual guide to build a nutrient-dense plate:

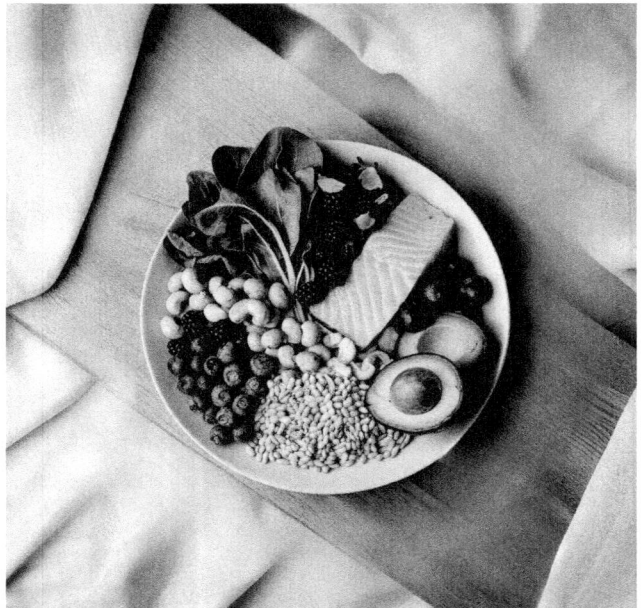

- **Proteins:** Fill a quarter of your plate with lean proteins, like grilled chicken or chickpeas.
- **Whole grains:** Use another quarter for whole grains, such as quinoa or brown rice.
- **Leafy greens and vegetables:** Half your plate should be colorful vegetables and leafy greens.
- **Healthy fats:** Add a small portion of healthy fats, like a quarter of an avocado or a handful of nuts.

This template offers a simple way to ensure that you're getting a balance of nutrients, supporting your fasting practice and overall health. By focusing on nutrient density and variety, you can create meals that taste good and make you feel good.

MEALS FOR HORMONAL HEALTH AND METABOLIC BOOST

I used to start my day with a cup of coffee (or three). But I would invariably feel worse as the morning went on. Now I start my day with a full cup of water and don't have my coffee until midmorning. This is ideal since we all wake up dehydrated, and drinking caffeine immediately doesn't help.

I follow that up with a creamy avocado-and-spinach smoothie at noon or twelve thirty. And this isn't just any smoothie. It's packed with healthy fats and iron that nourish your body from the inside out. Avocado brings a wealth of monounsaturated fats, which are fantastic for maintaining hormone balance, while spinach delivers a punch of iron, essential for energy—especially if you're feeling fatigued. Blend with some almond milk and a handful of blueberries for a touch of sweetness and antioxidants. This kind of breakfast sets you up for the day, fuels you with sustained energy, and keeps those hunger pangs at bay.

As the day progresses, you will want to focus on having a lunch that satisfies and supports your hormonal balance. A quinoa salad tossed with nuts and seeds does precisely that. Quinoa is a complete protein that provides all the essential amino acids your body needs. When paired with nuts and seeds, like almonds and chia, this salad becomes a powerhouse of phytoestrogens. These natural compounds mimic estrogen in the body and help balance hormones. This is particularly beneficial if you're navigating the complexities of menopause. Add a mix of colorful vegetables—think bell peppers and cherry tomatoes—to bring in an array of vitamins and minerals.

When it comes to dinner, consider a spicy lentil soup that not only delights your palate but also revs up your metabolism. Lentils are an excellent plant-based protein and fiber source that promotes satiety and digestive health. By incorporating metabolism-boosting spices like cayenne pepper and turmeric, you're adding flavor and encouraging your body to burn calories more efficiently. Spices have long been celebrated for their thermogenic properties, which can slightly increase your body temperature and metabolism. This soup can be a comforting end to the day, warming your body and soul while supporting your metabolic functions.

Cooking with seasonal and accessible ingredients supports your health and connects you to the rhythms of the Earth. Seasonal produce tends to be fresher, more flavorful, and packed with nutrients. For example, in the fall, you might incorporate roasted butternut squash into your meals, while in the summer, fresh berries could be your go-to snack. Shopping at local markets can inspire you to try new ingredients and experiment with your meals. This practice enriches your diet and supports local farmers, creating community and sustainability in your eating habits.

To preserve all the nutrients in your meals, consider cooking methods that maintain their integrity. Gentle steaming and sautéing help retain vitamins and minerals. Steaming broccoli or carrots keeps them crisp and bright, locking in flavor and nutrients. Sautéing, on the other hand, involves cooking foods quickly over high heat, enhancing flavors while keeping the nutritional value intact. Whether preparing a simple stir-fry or a more elaborate dish, these methods can elevate your meals, ensuring that you get the most out of every bite.

CLEAN FASTING: WHAT TO CONSUME DURING FASTING WINDOWS

The term *clean fasting* might sound like the latest health trend, but it's actually a straightforward practice. It involves abstaining from any food or drink that could interfere with the benefits of fasting. The idea is to give your body a true rest from digestion, allowing it to focus on repair and rejuvenation.

During clean fasting, water becomes your best friend. Staying hydrated is crucial, as it helps maintain your body's functions and supports the detoxification that occurs while you fast. You might be surprised at how much a simple glass of water fills you up and keeps hunger at bay. Black coffee and plain tea are also acceptable, offering a comforting ritual without adding calories. These beverages can even boost metabolism slightly, giving you a gentle nudge of energy during your fasting hours.

Hydration plays a pivotal role in the success of your fasting regimen. When you fast, your body shifts gears, and staying hydrated helps it transition smoothly. Water is essential for keeping your skin looking healthy, your digestion running smoothly, and your mind clear. But plain water is only one of many options. Consider adding a slice of lemon or a splash of apple cider vinegar. These add-ins enhance flavor and help maintain your electrolyte balance. Herbal teas, such as peppermint or chamomile, are another alternative. They're soothing and make hydration feel less monotonous. Electrolytes are key during fasting, as they help regulate muscle function and nerve impulses. You can make a simple homemade electrolyte by adding a pinch of salt and a squeeze of lemon to your water.

Even with the best intentions, fasting can sometimes present challenges. Hunger pangs, for instance, are a common hurdle. Understanding that some hunger is normal, especially when you first start fasting, can help you manage it. Instead of reaching for a snack, try engaging in a mindful activity. Deep breathing exercises, light stretching, or even a walk outside can distract you and help you refocus. Sometimes, hunger isn't actually about needing food—it can be about needing a change of scenery or a moment of calm. If you find your mind wandering to thoughts of food, consider journaling or meditating for a few minutes. These practices can ground you and remind you of your fasting goals. I use time blocking on my calendar to make sure I schedule time during the late morning, when hunger might sneak into my consciousness.

If you enjoy a bit of flavor, apple cider vinegar is a wonderful addition to your fasting routine. A small amount, diluted in water, can aid digestion and curb appetite. It's a staple in the fasting community for its purported benefits, including how it supports gut health. However, it's important to remember that moderation is key. Too much of anything, even something healthful, can be counterproductive. Start with a teaspoon in a glass of water and see how your body responds.

Interactive Element: Mindful Fasting Checklist

- **Hydration goal:** Aim for at least eight cups of water, adjusting for activity level and climate.
- **Mindful activities:** List three quick activities that distract you from hunger (such as a five-minute walk, deep breathing, or listening to music).
- **Fasting beverage options:** Keep a variety of teas and coffee options available to maintain interest and satisfaction.
- **Journaling prompt:** Reflect on how you feel during fasting. What emotions or thoughts arise? How do they impact your fasting experience?

Focusing on clean fasting and incorporating these mindful practices can enhance your fasting success and make the experience more enjoyable.

DIRTY FASTING: A FLEXIBLE APPROACH

A great way to ease into fasting is through what is referred to as dirty fasting. Unlike clean fasting, which strictly avoids calories, dirty fasting offers a bit more flexibility. It allows for low-calorie drinks, bone broth, or that little touch of cream in your coffee. This approach makes fasting feel more approachable and less intimidating, offering an easier way to ease in without the pressure of a strict fasting routine. It's a realistic option if you're looking for balance while adapting to a fasting lifestyle.

If you're new to fasting, dirty fasting can serve as a helpful bridge. It eases you into the practice without the immediate shock of strict calorie restriction, allowing your body to gradually adapt to fasting's demands. This gentler method can particularly benefit women over forty, as our bodies often respond better to incremental changes. By incorporating small amounts of calories, you may find it easier to extend your fasting periods, then eventually transition to longer fasting windows if desired. The key is to listen to your body and find a rhythm that aligns with your lifestyle and health goals.

One of the most significant benefits of dirty fasting is its ability to help curb hunger and cravings. We all know those moments when hunger hits unexpectedly, and the thought of enduring it seems unbearable. With dirty fasting, you can include small, low-calorie snacks that help keep these feelings in check without fully breaking your fast. Bone broth, for instance, is a popular choice. It's nourishing and provides electrolytes, which are imperative while fasting. Similarly, a small amount of cream in your coffee can provide just enough satisfaction to keep you going. Allowing these minor indulgences can make it easier to stick with your fasting regimen.

The mental aspect of fasting can often be the most challenging. Many people struggle with the idea of abstaining from food, particularly when surrounded by tempting options. Dirty fasting offers a psychological break, allowing you to enjoy a few comforts without feeling like you're completely off track. This flexibility can alleviate the mental burden of fasting, making it feel less like a chore and more like a manageable lifestyle choice. It's about finding a balance that works for you and respects your body's needs while still reaping the benefits of fasting.

Dirty fasting aims to create a practice that feels attainable and realistic. It's about embracing life's imperfections and realizing that small adjustments can still lead to significant progress. If dirty fasting helps you be consistent with your fasting, then it's serving its purpose. Remember, the journey to health is personal, and there is no one-size-fits-all approach. Embrace the flexibility dirty fasting offers and let it guide you toward a healthier, more energetic you.

KETO-FRIENDLY AND HORMONE-FEASTING MEALS

Have you ever wondered why some people swear by keto when it comes to fasting? With its low-carb, high-fat approach, the keto diet can be a powerful companion to intermittent fasting. When you reduce carbohydrate intake, your body enters a state called ketosis, where it burns fat for fuel instead of glucose. This increased fat-burning can amplify the effects of fasting, making it easier to shed those stubborn pounds and maintain steady energy levels throughout the day. This approach can be particularly beneficial for many women over forty, as it aligns with the body's natural tendency to store fat during hormonal changes.

Hormone-feasting give you a chance to indulge in meals that satisfy and support hormonal health. This might include a perfectly cooked salmon served alongside crisp, tender asparagus. This meal is rich in omega-3 fatty acids and phytoestrogens, which help balance hormones and support heart health. Salmon provides essential nutrients that can reduce inflammation, while asparagus offers a dose of fiber and vitamins. For breakfast or brunch, consider an egg frittata packed with leafy greens, like kale or spinach. Eggs provide high-quality protein and are rich in iron, which is essential for producing energy. The greens add a burst of nutrients and flavor, making this dish both nourishing and delicious.

Balancing keto with fasting requires a strategic approach, particularly when it comes to carbohydrates. Carb cycling involves alternating between high-carb and low-carb days. This technique can prevent the body from adapting too much to a low-carb diet, avoiding plateaus and maintaining metabolic flexibility. On high-carb days, you might enjoy sweet potatoes or quinoa, which give your body the energy it needs for more intense activities. On low-carb days, stick to your keto-friendly options to stay in a fat-burning state. This balance allows you to enjoy the benefits of both keto and fasting without feeling deprived.

However, it's important to navigate the potential pitfalls of combining keto with fasting. One common mistake is neglecting nutrient diversity. While keto focuses on fats and proteins, it's crucial to get a variety of nutrients. A diet overly rich in fatty meats and dairy with little else can lead to deficiencies. Make sure you eat a wide range of vegetables, seeds, and nuts to cover your nutritional bases. Another issue is dehydration, as low-carb diets can lead to a loss of electrolytes. So drink plenty of water and consider electrolyte supplements.

Personalization is key as you explore these dietary strategies. Listen to your body and adjust as needed. Not every approach works for everyone, and that's okay. Experiment with different meals, pay attention to how you feel and enjoy discovering what works best for you. The goal is to find a harmonious balance that supports your health and enhances your fasting experience.

MEAL TIMING: SYNCHRONIZING WITH CIRCADIAN RHYTHMS

Have you ever noticed that your energy levels seem to shift throughout the day, sometimes leaving you feeling alert and other times craving a nap? This natural ebb and flow is guided by your circadian rhythm, an internal clock that influences various biological processes. By aligning your meal times with these rhythms, you can enhance your fasting and overall health.

The concept of circadian rhythm fasting suggests consuming meals during daylight hours, which can help regulate your hormones and metabolism. Daylight eating means you time your meals to coincide with your body's natural energy peaks—typically in the morning and midafternoon. This approach can help stabilize blood sugar, improve digestion, and enhance your ability to burn calories efficiently.

Meal timing plays a crucial role in weight management and metabolic health. A nourishing breakfast can boost your metabolism, kick-start your energy production, and set you up for success. A hearty meal in the morning can help regulate hunger hormones, keeping you satisfied until your next meal. This could include lots of whole grains, protein, and healthy fats. These components work together to fuel your morning activities and prevent mid-morning energy slumps. By planning your meals around your body's natural rhythms, you create a harmonious balance that supports weight management and overall well-being.

A practical example of circadian rhythm fasting might involve an early dinner, completed before sunset. This allows your body to enter its fasting phase aligned with the natural decrease in energy use as evening approaches. This aids digestion and supports better sleep, as your body isn't focused on metabolizing a late meal. For instance, you might have dinner around six p.m., giving yourself ample time to digest before bedtime.

Synchronizing meals with your body's clock isn't just a modern concept. It's deeply rooted in cultural traditions worldwide. The Mediterranean diet, for example, is known for its health benefits and is a shining example of how you can naturally integrate meal timing into everyday life. This dietary pattern emphasizes enjoying leisurely meals earlier in the evening and even during daylight hours. It features fresh fruits and vegetables, whole grains, lean proteins, and healthy fats. This approach supports circadian rhythms and encourages mindful eating practices.

Incorporating circadian rhythm fasting into your lifestyle requires some planning, but the benefits are well worth the effort. By paying attention to when you eat—not just what you eat—you can optimize your body's natural processes and support overall health. This approach may lead to improved energy levels, better digestion, and more effective weight management, making it a powerful tool in your fasting tool kit. If you embrace the opportunity to sync your meals with your body's rhythms, you may find new levels of stamina and well-being.

BALANCING MACRONUTRIENTS FOR OPTIMAL FASTING

Navigating the world of nutrition can sometimes feel like a balancing act, especially when it comes to macronutrients. Proteins, fats, and carbohydrates—the three pillars of nutrition—all play their own unique role in supporting a successful fasting lifestyle.

Proteins: Often considered the building blocks of the body, proteins are crucial for maintaining muscle mass, which is particularly important as we age. Lean meats, such as chicken and turkey, provide high-quality protein without excess fat. For plant-based options, lentils and chickpeas offer a robust protein profile, making them versatile staples in any diet. These proteins keep your muscles strong and support recovery, providing the foundation you need during fasting periods.

Fats: Often misunderstood, fats are a fundamental source of energy and contribute to a feeling of fullness. The healthy fats found in avocados, nuts, and seeds can help you feel fuller longer, reducing the temptation to snack between meals. These fats also support hormone production, especially for women navigating hormonal changes. By consuming a variety of healthy fats, you create a meal plan that satisfies hunger and supports overall well-being. Imagine a salad topped with sliced avocado and a sprinkle of delicious and nourishing walnuts.

Carbohydrates: Carbohydrates, the body's preferred energy source, also play an important role. While it's easy to view carbs as the enemy, they are essential for brain function and mood regulation. Complex carbohydrates, such as those found in whole grains and sweet potatoes, release energy slowly and help stabilize blood sugar levels. This can improve your mood and help you focus, as carbs help regulate serotonin, the neurotransmitter linked to happiness and relaxation. By choosing the right types of carbohydrates, you can fuel your body effectively without the spikes and crashes associated with refined sugars.

Finding the right balance between these macronutrients can make all the difference. A typical macronutrient distribution is 40 percent carbohydrates, 30 percent protein, and 30 percent fats. This balance gives you the energy you need while providing nutrients for muscle maintenance and satiety. However, it's important to remember that these ratios aren't set in stone. Your needs may vary based on your activity level, age, and specific health goals. If you're more active, you can support muscle recovery and growth by eating more protein. It's all about listening to your body and making adjustments to suit your lifestyle.

One of the beautiful things about macronutrients is their impact on hormonal health. Properly balanced meals can help balance your hormones, reducing fatigue and mood swings. By ensuring a steady intake of these macronutrients, you provide your body with the tools it needs to function optimally during fasting and beyond.

As you explore the world of macronutrients, remember that personalizing your approach is key. Experiment with different ratios and observe how your body responds. You might find that you need a bit more protein or carbs on days when you're more physically active. The goal is to see what works best for you, supporting your fasting goals while enhancing your overall health.

4

ENHANCING ENERGY AND MENTAL CLARITY

"Eat with intention and presence. Every meal is an opportunity to nourish not just your body, but your mind." — Thich Nhat Hanh

Let's paint a picture: It's three p.m., and you're fighting the urge to guzzle another cup of coffee just to make it through the rest of the day.

Sound familiar? I know it does to me!

You're not alone. Many women over forty experience an energy roller coaster. Fatigue hits like clockwork, making even simple tasks feel monumental. This isn't just about getting older. It's a reflection of deeper changes occurring in your body.

Hormonal shifts, particularly those related to perimenopause and menopause, can leave you feeling drained. Estrogen and progesterone, the two main hormones, play a crucial role in regulating energy levels. As they fluctuate, they can disrupt your sleep and mood, leading to persistent fatigue. But it's not just hormones. Nutritional gaps can exacerbate the situation. Without the proper nutrients, your body struggles to maintain energy, leaving you feeling perpetually worn out.

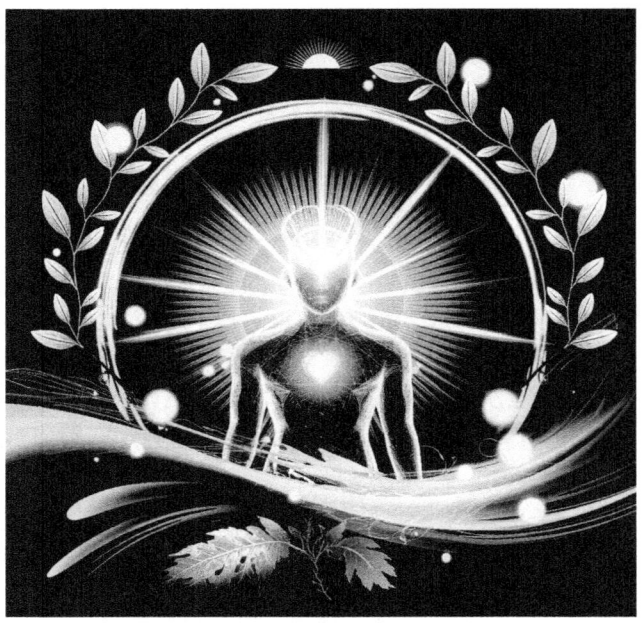

Intermittent fasting might just be the key to unlocking a more energetic version of yourself. It works by enhancing metabolic efficiency, essentially teaching your body to use energy more wisely. During fasting, your body switches from burning glucose to burning fat, a more stable form of energy. This shift can help stabilize your blood sugar and reduce the dramatic energy dips you might be accustomed to. By giving your digestive system a break, fasting allows your body to focus on repair and rejuvenation, which can give you noticeably more energy. It's like hitting the reset button, allowing you to start fresh each day with renewed vigor.

However, diving headfirst into fasting can lead to fatigue, especially if your body isn't accustomed to it. To avoid this, consider a gradual approach.

Start with shorter fasting windows and slowly increase them as your body adapts. This can prevent the energy dips that often accompany sudden dietary changes.

Another strategy is to incorporate rest days into your routine.

These aren't days off from fasting but rather days when you focus on nourishing your body with nutrient-dense foods and plenty of rest. By balancing energy expenditure with recovery, you ensure that fasting remains a sustainable part of your lifestyle.

> **Mary Jane's Story:** When my friend Mary Jane hit her mid-forties, she found herself constantly tired and struggling to keep up with her daily responsibilities. She decided to try intermittent fasting, starting with a simple twelve-hour fast. Within weeks, she began to notice a difference. Her energy levels started to stabilize, and she no longer needed that afternoon caffeine fix. Mary Jane's story shows the potential of fasting in combating fatigue. It's not just about what you eat but when you eat and how you allow your body the time it needs to restore itself.

Interactive Element: Energy Journal Prompt: Consider keeping an energy journal to track your progress as you incorporate fasting. Each day, jot down how you feel before, during, and after your eating windows. Note any changes in energy levels, mood, or focus. Over time, you'll likely start to see patterns emerge, providing insight into what works best for you. Reflect on these entries weekly to make any necessary adjustments to your fasting routine. This helps you stay accountable and empowers you to make informed decisions about your health.

BOOSTING MENTAL CLARITY AND FOCUS

When I was in my twenties and thirties, I used to wake up in the morning not only rested but mentally sharp. My thoughts were clear, and my focus was unshakeable. This is the kind of mental clarity that intermittent fasting can help you achieve in your forties and beyond.

As we age, brain fog and lapses in concentration become more common, often leaving us searching for words or struggling to focus on tasks.

Fasting, however, offers a unique approach to enhancing brain function. One of the key cognitive benefits of fasting is its ability to stabilize blood sugar. When your blood sugar is stable, your concentration improves, and you can focus on tasks more easily. This stability helps you stay sharp and alert, making it easier to tackle the day's challenges.

Fasting also has neuroprotective effects, which refers to its ability to protect nerve cells (neurons) from damage, degeneration, or dysfunction, thus supporting overall cognitive health. During fasting, your brain shifts to using ketones—byproducts of fat breakdown —as a primary fuel source. Ketones are more efficient than glucose, and they provide your brain with a steady supply of energy. This shift can lead to improved mental acuity and clear brain fog, leaving you feeling more mentally agile. Scientific studies support these benefits, showing that fasting can enhance memory and cognitive function. Research has found that intermittent fasting promotes the growth of new neurons and increases brain-derived neurotrophic factor (BDNF), a protein linked to learning and memory.[1]

To maximize these cognitive benefits, consider incorporating brain exercises into your routine. Just like physical exercise strengthens your muscles, mental exercises can sharpen your brain. Doing puzzles and crosswords, or even learning a new skill, can stimulate your brain and enhance focus. Incorporate short bursts of these activities throughout your day to keep your mind engaged and sharp. Staying hydrated is also crucial for mental clarity. Even mild dehydration can affect your mood and cognitive function, so be sure to drink plenty of water throughout the day. Proper hydration

---

1. Alby Elias, Noushad Padinjakara, and Nicola T. Lautenschlager, "Effects of intermittent fasting on cognitive health and Alzheimer's disease," *Oxford Academic* 81 no. 9 (2023): 1225-33.

supports brain function and helps maintain concentration, allowing you to stay focused and alert.

The cognitive benefits of fasting are backed by scientific research. Studies have shown that fasting can improve memory and cognitive function, providing scientific validation for what many people experience firsthand. For example, research published in the journal *Neurobiology of Aging* found that intermittent fasting can enhance synaptic plasticity, which is crucial for learning and memory.[2] These findings confirm that fasting is more than just a dietary practice. It's a powerful tool for supporting brain health.

MINDFULNESS PRACTICES TO ENHANCE FASTING BENEFITS

Approach your fasting routine not just as a means to an end but as a way to cultivate awareness and presence in your life. This is where mindfulness comes into play. Mindfulness in fasting is about homing in on the experience, paying attention to how your body feels, and making conscious choices that align with your well-being. It's about being present in the now, appreciating each aspect of your fasting routine, and recognizing the subtle signals your body sends.

When you practice mindful eating, you become aware of the flavors and textures of your food, the sensations of hunger and fullness, and the emotions attached to eating. This heightened awareness can transform your relationship with food, making each meal a deliberate and thoughtful experience. By savoring each bite and acknowledging its nourishment, you create a more intentional and fulfilling relationship with your diet.

Mindfulness can also have a profound impact on energy and clarity. By focusing your attention on the present moment, you can

---

2. Eunyoung Bang, Annette S. Fincher, Sophie Nader, David A. Murchison, and William H. Griffith, "Late-Onset, Short-Term Intermittent Fasting Reverses Age-Related Changes in Calcium Buffering and Inhibitory Synaptic Transmission in Mouse Basal Forebrain Neurons," *The Journal of Neuroscience* 42 no. 6 (2022): 1020-34.

stabilize your energy levels and improve your focus. Mindful practices, such as meditation or deep breathing exercises, help you stay grounded, reducing the mental clutter that often accompanies a busy life. When your mind is clear, you can channel your energy more effectively, ensuring that it supports your daily activities rather than hindering them. This clarity can enhance your productivity, allowing you to tackle tasks with renewed vigor and intention. The simple act of pausing and centering yourself can prevent energy drains and keep you on track.

Incorporating mindfulness into your fasting routine is easier than you might think. Consider setting aside time for meditation sessions, during which you engage in guided breathing exercises that calm your mind and body. These sessions can be as short as five minutes, offering a moment of tranquility amidst the chaos of daily life. Focus on your breath, allowing each inhale and exhale to anchor you in the present.

Alternatively, try keeping a gratitude journal. During your fasting periods, take a few minutes to reflect on what you're grateful for. This practice can shift your perspective, helping you appreciate the small joys in life and fostering contentment. By combining meditation and gratitude, you create a balanced approach that supports both your mental and emotional well-being.

Kristen's Story: Kristen, a busy mom of two, found herself overwhelmed by the demands of work and family. Initially skeptical, she decided to incorporate mindfulness into her fasting routine. She began each day with a short meditation, focusing on her breath and setting intentions for the day. During her fasting window, she wrote down what she was grateful for, noting moments of joy and appreciation. Over time, Kristen noticed a marked improvement in her energy and clarity. The mental fog lifted, and she felt more in tune with her body and mind. Fasting became not just a dietary practice but a holistic approach to living more mindfully.

Kristen's story underscores the potential of mindfulness to enhance fasting benefits. When you integrate mindfulness into your fasting routines, you can experience a deeper connection to your body and greater well-being. Mindfulness fosters an awareness that extends beyond fasting and influences other aspects of life. By cultivating this awareness, you can create a more balanced and harmonious lifestyle that supports your physical, mental, and emotional health. Mindfulness invites you to slow down, savor each moment, and find joy in the present, transforming fasting from a simple practice into a meaningful experience.

OVERCOMING BRAIN FOG WITH NUTRIENT SUPPORT

Have you ever been sitting at your desk, trying to focus on the task at hand, but your mind feels like it's wading through the fog? You're not alone. Many women over forty experience brain fog, a frustrating state of mental cloudiness that can make even simple tasks seem insurmountable. This isn't just a phase. It's often rooted in nutritional deficiencies that have snuck up over the years.

As our bodies change, so do our nutritional needs. When these aren't met, cognitive function can suffer. B vitamins, for example, are crucial for maintaining energy and cognitive function. They play a key role in producing neurotransmitters, the brain's chemical messengers, which are essential for clear thinking and memory. A lack of these vitamins can leave you feeling mentally sluggish.

Antioxidants are another central component. They protect brain cells from damage caused by free radicals, which can accelerate aging and cognitive decline. By fortifying your diet with these nutrients, you can help ward off the fog and bring clarity back to your day.

So, how can you give your brain the boost it needs? Start by including in your diet foods rich in B vitamins and antioxidants:

- **Leafy greens**, such as spinach and kale, are packed with these nutrients and are easy to incorporate into meals.

- **Berries**, particularly blueberries, are another powerhouse. They're loaded with antioxidants that have been shown to enhance communication between brain cells, improving memory and cognitive function.
- **Omega-3** supplements can also be beneficial. Found naturally in fatty fish, like salmon, these healthy fats are essential for brain health, supporting cell membrane integrity and reducing inflammation. If fish isn't your thing, consider an omega-3 supplement to ensure that you're getting enough of this crucial nutrient.

Creating brain-boosting meal plans doesn't have to be complicated. Aim for balanced meals that incorporate a variety of brain-healthy foods.

- **Breakfast:** Consider an omelet with spinach and tomatoes paired with a side of fresh berries. This meal provides a good mix of protein, healthy fats, and antioxidants to start your day on the right foot.
- **Lunch:** How about a hearty salad with mixed greens, walnuts, and grilled chicken with olive oil and lemon juice? Walnuts are another excellent source of omega-3s, and when combined with the healthy fats in olive oil, they create a satisfying and nutritious meal.
- **Dinner:** Feature grilled salmon alongside broccoli and quinoa, offering a balance of proteins, healthy fats, and carbohydrates.

This meal plan ensures that you're nourishing both your body and mind, setting the stage for improved focus and mental clarity.

Planning these meals doesn't have to be a chore. Think of it as an opportunity to explore new recipes and flavors. Start by setting aside time each week to plan your meals. Consider batch cooking or prepping ingredients in advance to make mealtimes easier. This can help you avoid the temptation of less nutritious convenience foods when you're short on time.

Experiment with spices and herbs to add flavor without extra calories. Turmeric, for example, has powerful anti-inflammatory properties and can be a flavorful addition to soups and stews. By focusing on nutrient-dense foods and embracing variety, you can create meals that are both delicious and beneficial for your brain health.

Finally, remember that small changes can make a big difference. You don't have to overhaul your entire diet overnight. Start by incorporating a few brain-healthy foods into your meals and gradually build from there. Pay attention to how these changes affect your mental clarity and energy levels. You might be surprised at how quickly you notice a difference. As you continue to nourish your brain with the right nutrients, you'll likely find that the fog begins to lift and is replaced by a newfound focus and clarity.

ENERGY-BOOSTING FOODS FOR FASTING DAYS

Waking up to a day full of possibilities is invigorating, yet it's not always easy to maintain that initial energy surge throughout your fasting days. The secret often lies in the fuel you choose.

Nutrient-dense foods can play a pivotal role in sustaining energy, keeping you active and focused as the day unfolds. It's not just about eating but choosing what will serve your body best. Complex carbohydrates and proteins are your allies here. They provide long-lasting energy, slowly releasing glucose into your bloodstream and preventing those dreaded energy crashes. Consider starting your day with oatmeal sprinkled with almonds or a breakfast of eggs and whole-grain toast. These meals combine the slow-release energy of carbs with the muscle-supporting power of protein, giving you a balanced start.

When you think of high-energy foods, quinoa, and sweet potatoes should top your list. Quinoa, a complete protein, is packed with essential amino acids, making it an excellent choice for vegetarians and meat-eaters alike. Its versatility means you can enjoy it in salads, as a side dish, or even in breakfast bowls.

Sweet potatoes, on the other hand, are rich in fiber and vitamin A, increasing your energy levels and overall health. Their natural sweetness makes them a delightful addition to any meal, whether baked, mashed, or roasted. Including these foods in your diet can help keep your energy reserves steady, even on fasting days.

Strategically timing your meals can further enhance your energy levels. Pre-fasting meals are crucial; they set the stage for how you'll feel throughout your fasting period. Aim to consume a meal rich in complex carbs and proteins about an hour before your fasting window begins. This gives your body time to digest and absorb nutrients, providing a stable energy source as you transition into fasting. For example, a salad with grilled chicken, quinoa, and a variety of colorful vegetables can be both satisfying and energizing. Pair this with a piece of fruit or a handful of nuts, and you'll be well-prepared for your fasting hours.

Simple recipes can be a lifesaver when you're on the go and need a quick energy boost. Homemade energy bars—made with oats, nuts, and a touch of honey—are a convenient snack to keep on hand. They require minimal prep, and you can tailor them to your taste by adding dried fruits or seeds. I make sure to always have one on hand and include it in my carry-on when I travel.

Smoothies, too, offer a quick and delicious way to maintain energy. Blend a banana, a scoop of protein powder, a handful of spinach, and a splash of almond milk for a refreshing and revitalizing drink. These options are nutritious and easy to make. Plus, they give you the fuel you need, no matter what your day holds.

Incorporating these energy-boosting foods and strategies into your routine can make a significant difference in how you feel during fasting days. By focusing on nutrient density and meal timing, you can create a foundation for sustained energy and overall well-being. Whether you're preparing a hearty meal or grabbing a quick snack, remember that your choices have the power to transform your energy levels and enhance your fasting experience.

MAINTAINING ENERGY CONSISTENCY IN DAILY LIFE

Have you ever woken up feeling refreshed, ready to tackle the day, only to find that by midafternoon, your energy has dwindled? This scenario is all too common, especially as we age. While diet plays a crucial role in maintaining energy, lifestyle habits are equally significant.

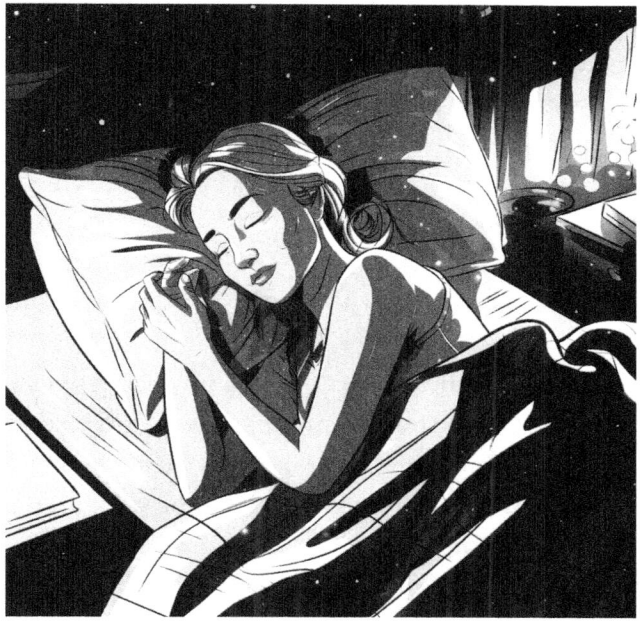

Get Better Sleep

Sleep quality is paramount. Restful sleep allows your body to repair and rejuvenate, setting the foundation for a productive day.

Developing a consistent sleep routine can be beneficial. Aim for seven to nine hours of sleep each night, and try to maintain a regular sleep-wake schedule, even on weekends. Creating a calming bedtime routine, such as reading or listening to soothing music, can signal to your body that it's time to wind down. Avoid screens before bed, as the blue light can interfere with your natural sleep cycle.

Manage Your Stress

Stress management is another critical factor. Chronic stress drains energy, leaving you feeling fatigued and overwhelmed. Incorporating relaxation techniques into your daily routine can help mitigate stress. Consider trying yoga, meditation, or deep breathing exercises. They promote relaxation and help clear your mind, allowing you to approach tasks with renewed focus and energy. Even taking a few minutes throughout the day to pause and breathe deeply can make a significant difference. By managing stress, you create a calmer and more balanced environment, which supports consistent energy levels.

Get Active

Short breaks and physical activity are invaluable when it comes to maintaining energy throughout the day. Sitting for prolonged periods can sap your energy, making you tired and less productive. So get moving! Take short breaks to stretch or walk around. Even a five-minute walk can increase circulation and boost energy. If possible, stand while working or alternate between sitting and standing. This simple change can improve your posture and reduce fatigue. Regular physical activity, such as walking, dancing, or swimming, is good for your heart. Plus, it promotes energy consistency, which helps boost natural energy levels and keep them balanced and reliable. The key is finding activities you enjoy and making them a regular part of your routine.

Hydrate, Hydrate, Hydrate

Hydration is often overlooked but is essential for maintaining energy since dehydration can lead to fatigue and decreased focus. If you're dehydrated, you can be extra tired and have trouble concentrating. Make it a habit to drink water throughout the day, aiming for at least eight cups. Start your day with a glass of water to kick-start hydration, and keep a water bottle handy as a reminder to sip regularly.

If plain water doesn't appeal to you, try infusing it with fruits or herbs for a refreshing twist. Staying hydrated helps regulate body temperature and supports all bodily functions, ensuring that you have the energy to tackle daily tasks.

A balanced lifestyle is the cornerstone of sustained energy. The interplay of diet, exercise, and wellness practices creates a harmonious environment for your body to thrive. When these elements are in sync, you experience more stable energy levels and improved well-being.

> **Suzanne's Story:** Consider Suzanne, a woman who struggled with fluctuating energy levels. By focusing on a balanced approach—prioritizing sleep, managing stress, and incorporating regular movement—she noticed a remarkable shift. She made small changes, such as going to bed at the same time every night, meditating daily, and taking a morning walk. Her energy stabilized, and she felt more capable of handling her daily responsibilities.

From prioritizing restful sleep and managing stress to staying hydrated and incorporating movement, these strategies work together to support consistent energy throughout the day. As you incorporate these practices into your routine, you may find a newfound sense of strength and balance.

MAKE A DIFFERENCE WITH YOUR REVIEW

> *"Never believe that a few caring people can't change the world. Indeed, it's the only thing that ever has."* — Margaret Mead

As someone who understands the unique challenges we face during this season of life, you know that finding reliable, practical advice isn't always easy. Your honest review would be invaluable in helping other women discover how intermittent fasting can work for them, especially during these important years when our bodies need extra care and attention.

If you've found value in this book—whether it's through the customizable fasting schedules, the hormone-balancing strategies, or the supportive community approach—would you consider sharing your experience? Your voice matters, and your review could encourage another woman to take that first step toward better health.

Here's what would be helpful to include in your review:

- How the book helped you understand intermittent fasting
- Which fasting approach worked best for your lifestyle
- Any positive changes you've noticed in your energy, sleep, or overall well-being
- How the supporting materials (meal plans, suggested schedules, or community resources) enhanced your journey

Remember, this isn't just about following a program. It's about embracing a sustainable approach to wellness that works for real women with real lives. Your authentic experience can make a meaningful difference, whether you're just starting or have been practicing for months.

To share your insights, simply scan the QR code below:

Every review helps build our community of strong, healthy women supporting each other through this journey. Thank you for helping other women as we all navigate this transitional time together.

5

SUSTAINABLE WEIGHT MANAGEMENT AND SYMPTOM RELIEF

"Small changes in diet and lifestyle can lead to remarkable improvements in health, happiness, and longevity" — Dr. Dean Ornish

If you've ever stood in front of your closet, trying on clothes that used to fit perfectly but were now snug and uncomfortable, you know that sinking feeling. It's a familiar scenario for many of us over forty as we navigate the intricacies of weight management amid hormonal shifts.

The quest for sustainable weight loss can feel daunting, especially when quick-fix diets promise rapid results but leave us in a cycle of disappointment. As we embark on this journey together, let's focus on a more balanced approach—one that promotes gradual, lasting change.

Sustainable weight loss isn't about drastic measures. It's about embracing slow, steady progress. It's like planting a seed and watching it grow; it takes time, patience, and care. Setting realistic goals is crucial. Rather than aiming to drop several dress sizes overnight, focus on achievable weekly targets. Perhaps it's shedding half a pound this week or simply incorporating more vegetables into your meals. These small, attainable goals build confidence and create momentum, transforming weight loss from a sprint into a marathon.

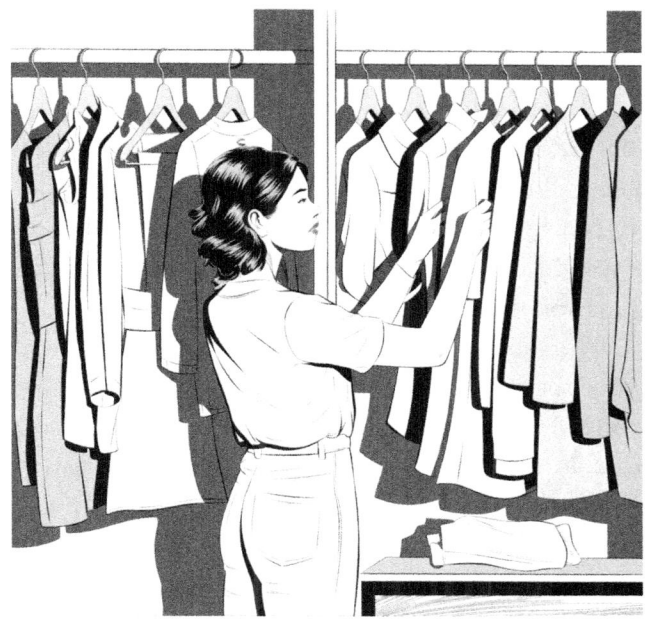

Incorporating small lifestyle changes can have a profound impact over time. Think about your daily habits. Are there areas where you can make minor adjustments? Maybe it's swapping sugary snacks for fruit or taking a short walk after dinner. These gradual changes, though seemingly insignificant, compound over time, leading to meaningful, sustainable weight loss. The beauty of this approach lies in its flexibility. You can tailor it to fit seamlessly into your life, respecting your body's needs and personal preferences.

Intermittent fasting plays a pivotal role in this sustainable approach, offering a framework for managing calories without depriving yourself. By designating specific eating windows, you naturally create a balance, allowing your body to rest and repair. This balance supports weight management by reducing calories in a controlled, healthy manner. Unlike restrictive diets that can leave you feeling deprived, fasting encourages mindful eating, making it easier to recognize true hunger signals and avoid overeating.

The dangers of extreme dieting cannot be overstated. While the allure of rapid weight loss is tempting, it often comes at a cost. Extreme dieting can lead to muscle loss, as the body breaks down muscle tissue for energy when it doesn't have adequate nutrition. This undermines weight loss efforts because it slows down metabolism and impacts overall health and energy. It's a cycle that's difficult to break. As a result, many women get frustrated and gain back any weight they lost. Prioritizing nutrition is key to avoiding these pitfalls and supporting long-term health.

Creating balanced meal plans is an essential component of keeping your weight where you want it to be. Start by focusing on portion control. Visualize your plate divided into sections: Half is filled with colorful vegetables, a quarter with lean protein, and the remaining quarter with whole grains. With this simple guide, you get a variety of nutrients, which supports both weight loss and overall well-being. Consider meal prepping to streamline this process, making it easier to stick to your plan even on busy days.

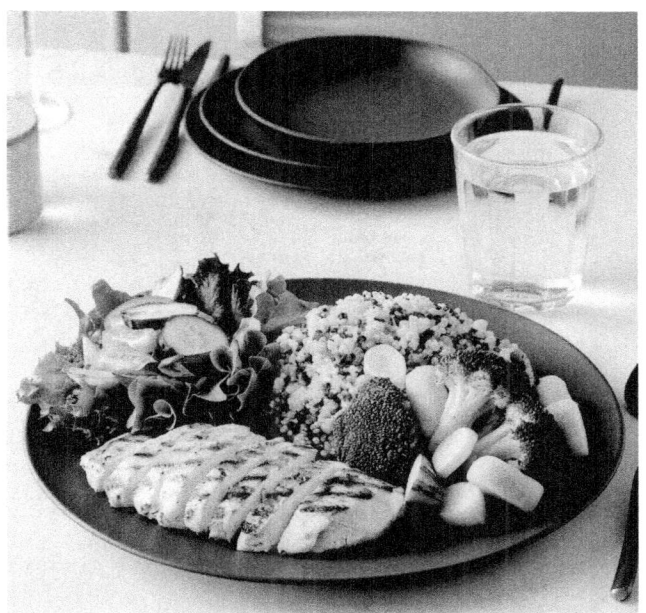

Interactive Element: Meal Planning Guide

- **Visualize your plate:** Draw a circle and divide it into sections for veggies, proteins, and grains. Use this guide when preparing meals.
- **Weekly meal prep:** Choose a day to plan your meals for the week. Prepare ingredients in advance to save time and reduce stress. See below an example of a 7-day meal plan.
- **Portion control:** Use measuring tools or your hand as a guide—palm-sized portions for proteins, fist-sized for grains, and an open hand for veggies.

16:8 INTERMITTENT FASTING 7-DAY MEAL PLAN

	Breakfast	Lunch	Dinner	Snack
Monday	Greek yogurt & berries	Grilled chicken breast with roasted sweet potato & broccoli	Baked salmon with lemon & asparagus	Handful of mixed nuts
Tuesday	Apple slices with almond butter	Quinoa salad with mixed greens & grilled chicken	Beef stir-fry with mixed vegetables & brown rice	Small bowl of berries
Wednesday	Carrot sticks with hummus	Tuna salad with mixed greens & avocado	Grilled chicken with a side of roasted Brussels sprouts & cauliflower	Small bowl of grapes
Thursday	Hard-boiled egg with cucumber slices	Grilled shrimp with a side of mixed vegetables & quinoa	Baked cod with steamed green beans	Handful of almonds
Friday	Peach slices with cottage cheese	Mixed greens salad with grilled chicken & cherry tomatoes	Beef chili with mixed veggies	Small bowl of blueberries
Saturday	Banana with almond butter	Spinach salad with grilled salmon & avocado	Baked chicken with roasted carrots	Handful of mixed nuts
Sunday	Trail mix with dried fruits & nuts	Grilled chicken breast with quinoa & mixed vegetables	Shrimp & vegetable stir-fry with brown rice	Small bowl of raspberries

By embracing these strategies and focusing on gradual, sustainable change, you can achieve weight loss that lasts and supports your health.

MANAGING HOT FLASHES THROUGH FASTING

Here is a typical scenario you may be familiar with: You're in the middle of a meeting or enjoying a quiet evening, and suddenly, a wave of heat engulfs you. Hot flashes, a common companion during menopause, can be both unexpected and uncomfortable. They can disrupt your day and your sleep, leaving you seeking relief wherever you can find it.

Intermittent fasting can be a part of the solution. By regulating your body's internal processes, fasting can help maintain a more stable body temperature, potentially reducing the frequency and intensity of these episodes. The key lies in hormonal regulation. As you fast, your body experiences a natural balance of hormones—particularly estrogen, which plays a significant role in managing body temperature. When estrogen levels fluctuate, the body can misinterpret these changes as overheating. That leads to those dreaded hot flashes. By stabilizing levels, fasting helps maintain a more consistent internal environment, reducing the likelihood of sudden and drastic temperature swings.

Dietary choices can further support this balance. Consider incorporating foods rich in phytoestrogens, such as flaxseeds, into your meals. Phytoestrogens are plant compounds that mimic estrogen in the body, offering a natural way to support hormonal balance. Flaxseeds, in particular, are easy to add to your diet. Sprinkle them on your morning oatmeal, blend them into smoothies, or mix them into a salad dressing. These small seeds pack a punch, offering phytoestrogens, fiber, and omega-3 fatty acids, which support overall health.

By making these simple dietary adjustments, you can enhance the benefits of fasting and support your hormones' proper functioning and balance, allowing your body to function smoothly, which, in turn, relieves symptoms.

Timing your fasting windows strategically can also help you manage hot flashes. Consider aligning your fasting periods to minimize nighttime symptoms. For many women, early-evening fasting is effective because it allows the body to enter a state of rest and repair well before bedtime. This timing can help reduce nighttime hot flashes, promoting better sleep and a more restful night. By ending your eating window earlier, you give your body ample time to digest and stabilize before night's cooler, restful hours. Imagine sipping a warm herbal tea as your last intake of the day, a soothing ritual that signals your body to transition into its fasting state.

> **Emily's Story:** When Emily was in her mid-fifties, she found herself wrestling with frequent, intense hot flashes that disrupted her work and sleep. After incorporating intermittent fasting and adjusting her eating window to end by seven p.m., she noticed a marked reduction in symptoms. Over time, her hot flashes became less frequent and less intense, allowing her to enjoy uninterrupted nights and more comfortable days. She also added more fiber and omega-3 fatty acids into her daily diet. Through journaling, she was able to identify what was working and adjust as necessary.

MOOD STABILIZATION WITH DIETARY ADJUSTMENTS

Before incorporating intermittent fasting into my lifestyle, I would be navigating my day, and out of nowhere, a wave of irritability or sadness would wash over me. It's not uncommon, especially during the hormonal shifts that occur after forty. But did you know that what you eat can play a significant role in how you feel?

Nutritional choices can profoundly impact your emotional well-being. Our brains rely on a delicate balance of chemicals to regulate mood, and diet is a crucial player in this balance. Foods rich in serotonin-boosting nutrients, like bananas and oats, can help maintain a more stable mood. Serotonin, often called the feel-good hormone, influences mood, sleep, and appetite. Incorporating serotonin-boosting foods into your diet can provide a natural lift and smooth out those emotional ups and downs.

To stabilize your mood even more, consider consuming more omega-3 fatty acids. These healthy fats, which are found abundantly in salmon, sardines, and walnuts, are known for their anti-inflammatory properties and ability to support brain health. Omega-3s can help modulate brain function, potentially alleviating depression and anxiety. By including these foods in your diet, you support your heart and brain health and nurture your emotional resilience. Imagine a delicious dinner of grilled salmon with a walnut-crusted topping paired with a side of roasted vegetables. These meals are satisfying and support a balanced mood.

Intermittent fasting can also help you manage mood swings. By offering your body consistent periods of rest from digestion, fasting helps regulate blood sugar, which can stabilize mood. When you fast, blood sugar levels have a chance to even out, reducing the spikes and crashes that can lead to irritability and mood swings. This stability creates calmness, allowing you to approach your day with a clearer head and more balanced emotions. It's about finding a rhythm that works for you, aligns with your lifestyle, and supports your mental health.

Incorporating mindfulness and relaxation techniques into your routine can smooth out your mood even more. Simple practices, such as breathing exercises, can offer instant calm and help you manage stress more effectively. When you feel tension rising, take a moment to pause and focus on your breath. Inhale deeply through your nose and count to four, allowing your belly to expand. Then hold for a count to two and exhale slowly through your mouth to a count to six. Repeat this process several times, feeling the tension melt away with each breath. These moments of mindfulness can be a reset button, grounding you and restoring a sense of peace. Pairing these practices with your dietary adjustments creates a comprehensive approach to managing your mood that supports both body and mind.

ADDRESSING BONE HEALTH AND OSTEOPOROSIS RISK

Think about the role your bones play in your daily life. They support you as you move, protect your organs, and store essential minerals. I was acutely aware of the importance of healthy and strong bones, as my mother developed osteoporosis in her sixties, which affected her overall health and well-being for the rest of her life.

As you move beyond menopause, the risk of osteoporosis—weak and brittle bones—increases significantly. This makes bone health a priority. It's crucial to pay attention to how you nourish your bones, ensuring that they remain strong and resilient.

Calcium and vitamin D stand out as the dynamic duo in this endeavor. Calcium is the primary building block of bone tissue, while vitamin D enhances calcium absorption, ensuring that your body utilizes it effectively. If you don't have enough of these nutrients, maintaining bone density becomes a challenge. Foods rich in calcium—like dairy products, leafy greens, and fortified plant milks—should become staples in your diet. For vitamin D, consider fatty fish (such as salmon), exposure to sunlight, and supplements if necessary.

Diet alone, however, is not enough to ensure bone health. Lifestyle modifications are equally important. Weight-bearing exercises are one of the most effective ways to maintain and improve bone density. Walking, jogging, and resistance training stimulate bone formation and slow down bone loss. These exercises don't have to be intense or time-consuming. A brisk walk around your neighborhood or simple resistance exercises with light weights can make a substantial difference. They benefit your bones and enhance muscle strength, balance, and coordination. By incorporating these exercises into your routine, you create a protective environment for your bones, reducing the risk of fractures and falls.

Intermittent fasting can play a supportive role in bone health, albeit indirectly. By improving metabolic health, fasting helps regulate insulin levels and reduce inflammation, both of which positively impact bone density. A balanced metabolism supports your body's natural repair processes, including those that maintain bone integrity. While fasting isn't a direct treatment for osteoporosis, its overall health benefits contribute to a stronger and more resilient body that's ready to support healthy bones. It's about creating an internal environment that gives your bones the nutrients and support they need.

Expert advice offers additional insights into maintaining bone health as you age. Nutritionists and healthcare professionals often recommend considering supplementation, especially if dietary intake falls short. Calcium and vitamin D supplements can be beneficial, particularly if you have dietary restrictions or limited sun exposure. It's essential to consult with a healthcare provider to determine the right dosage and ensure that supplementation complements your overall health plan and any prescription medicines you may be taking. They can guide you on the best forms of these nutrients, taking your individual needs and lifestyle into account. Remember, balance is key; too much calcium or vitamin D can lead to other health issues, such as kidney stones and digestive problems, so professional advice is invaluable.

PERSONALIZED FASTING ADJUSTMENTS

Intermittent fasting isn't a rigid plan but a flexible tool that you can adapt to your individual needs, especially as you navigate the changes that come with being over forty. This adaptability is where personalized fasting adjustments come into play. By tailoring fasting to your symptoms and lifestyle, you can enhance its benefits and create a routine that feels natural and sustainable.

Start by tracking your symptoms. Consider using a journal or app to monitor how you feel throughout your fasting journey. Note any patterns, such as increased hunger or fatigue at certain times, and use this information to adjust your fasting windows. If you find longer fasts challenging, shorter fasting windows can be a game-changer. Maybe a twelve-hour fast suits you better than the traditional 16:8 method. The key is to listen to your body and adjust as needed, allowing yourself the grace to experiment and find what feels right.

Feast days offer another layer of flexibility. On these days, you increase your calorie and nutrient intake, providing your body with the fuel it needs to recover and thrive. Feast days can be especially beneficial if you're feeling depleted or your body is signaling that it needs more nourishment. By incorporating these days into your routine, you maintain balance and prevent the fatigue that sometimes accompanies strict fasting schedules. It's about finding a rhythm that supports your energy and well-being.

Always remember that flexibility is crucial in any fasting practice. Your body's needs may change as you age, and it's important to adapt your fasting routine accordingly. Be open to adjusting your fasting windows, trying new foods, or incorporating different practices as your life evolves. This flexibility supports your physical health and fosters a positive relationship with fasting, making it a sustainable part of your lifestyle.

> **Nicci's Story:** Consider Nicci, a fifty-two-year-old who struggled with low energy and mood swings. She started fasting but found the traditional 16:8 method too demanding. Through trial and error, she discovered that a 14:10 fasting window, combined with regular feast days, worked best for her. This personalized approach allowed her to maintain her energy levels and improve her mood, demonstrating the power of tailoring fasting to your unique needs. Nicci's experience reveals the benefits of personalized fasting, showing that with patience and flexibility, you can create a practice that truly supports your health.

Personalizing your fasting practice is an opportunity to connect with your body and respond to its signals. By using tools, like symptom tracking, and embracing flexibility, you can create a fasting routine that aligns with your needs and lifestyle. Remember, the goal is not perfection but progress. Celebrate your successes and learn from setbacks, knowing each step brings you closer to a healthier, more balanced life.

BUILDING A WEIGHT MANAGEMENT ROUTINE

Creating a consistent routine is often like laying the foundation for a stable and long-lasting structure. It's the backbone of successful weight management, especially when you're juggling the demands of midlife. Integrating fasting and exercise into your daily schedule is crucial, not just for losing weight but for maintaining it.

Start by setting a daily schedule that includes specific times for eating and physical activity. This might mean designating a morning slot for a brisk walk or setting aside time for yoga in the afternoon. Consistency is key here; when your body knows what to expect, it adapts more readily, making it easier to stick to your goals.

Finding accountability partners can also be a game-changer. These are the people who cheer you on, keep you motivated, and sometimes give you the nudge you need when you're feeling less than enthusiastic. Maybe it's a friend who joins you for a walk or a family member who's on a similar health journey. Community groups, whether online or in person, offer a platform for shared experiences and mutual encouragement. Participating in local meetups or engaging in an online forum can provide the camaraderie you need. Sharing your challenges and triumphs with others can strengthen your resolve and inspire those around you.

Tracking your progress doesn't have to be a chore. With the plethora of digital trackers and apps available (such as Cronometer or MyFitnessPal, logging meals and exercise can become a seamless part of your routine. These tools provide insights into your habits, helping you identify patterns and areas for improvement. Whether you use a detailed app that monitors your calorie intake and expenditure or jot down your thoughts and progress in a simple journal, the goal is to keep a tangible record. Seeing your accomplishments on paper—or screen—can boost your confidence and help you stay on track.

Staying motivated is often easier said than done. That's why celebrating small victories is so important. Each step forward, no matter how small, is progress. Did you manage to stick to your fasting window all week? Celebrate it. Did you take the stairs instead of the elevator today? That's a win too. Recognizing and rewarding these achievements reinforces positive behavior and keeps you motivated to continue. Consider setting up a reward system for yourself—maybe a relaxing bath, a new book, or a treat that aligns with your health goals. These rewards remind you that your efforts are worthwhile and you're moving in the right direction.

As you build this routine, remember that flexibility is just as important as consistency. Life happens, and there will be days when things don't go as planned. When that happens, it's okay to adjust. The routine you establish should be a guide, not a rigid set of rules. Adaptability ensures that you can sustain your routine over the long term, allowing it to evolve with you. Listen to your body and your needs, and make changes when necessary. This approach supports weight management and contributes to a healthier, more balanced lifestyle overall.

6

LONGEVITY AND DISEASE PREVENTION

"The way you think, the way you behave, the way you eat, can influence your life by 30 to 50 years" — Deepak Chopra

As women, especially those of us over forty, we often find ourselves contemplating our long-term health and how best to preserve the energy and zest for life that we cherish. It's not just about adding years to our lives but bringing life to our years. Intermittent fasting emerges as a compelling ally in this quest, offering a pathway to longevity and enhanced life quality. This practice, backed by science, can extend our healthy years by reducing the risks of age-related diseases and supporting cellular health.

Studies have shown promising outcomes, particularly when it comes to reducing calories and how that can help us live longer. Research involving young males practicing fasting during Ramadan indicates that intermittent fasting can significantly lengthen lifespan by influencing nutrient-sensing pathways, enhancing the metabolic process, and activating autophagy, a cellular process through which cells break down their components. Studies have linked the activation of autophagy to longevity, and many proteins are involved in this process.[1] These findings suggest that fasting mimics the effects of caloric restriction, a well-researched method for promoting longevity. By reducing calorie intake without malnutrition, fasting triggers a cascade of beneficial effects that promote cellular repair and protect against age-related diseases.

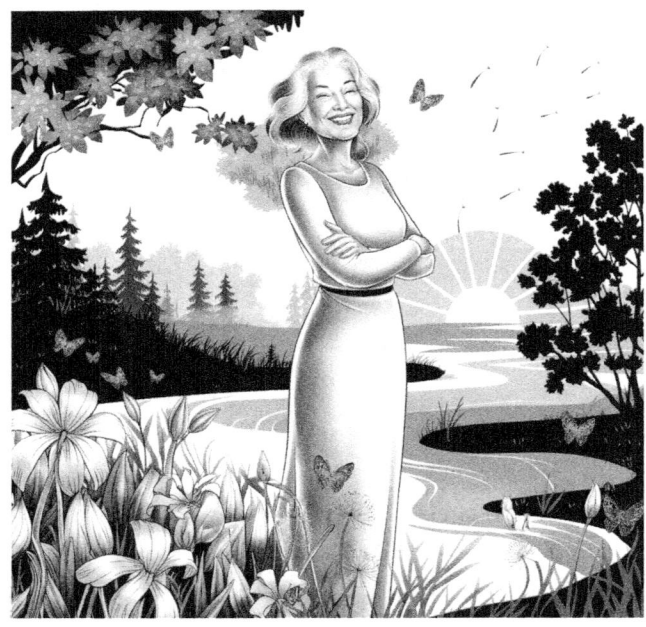

One of the most fascinating aspects of fasting is its ability to modulate the markers of aging. Biological markers, like telomeres—the protective caps at the ends of our chromosomes—play a crucial role in cellular aging. Fasting may help preserve telomere length, potentially slowing down the biological clock. Shortened telomeres are linked to a variety of age-related ailments, so maintaining their length through lifestyle interventions like fasting could be a game-

---

1. Anna Drangowska-Way, "Intermittent Fasting Induces Changes in Multiple Biomarkers," May 1, 2024, the Lifespan.io website, https://www.lifespan.io/news/intermittent-fasting-induces-changes-in-multiple-biomarkers.

changer. Additionally, fasting can reduce oxidative stress and inflammation, two key players in the aging process. By reducing oxidative damage and chronic inflammation, fasting supports a healthier cellular environment and fosters resilience against the wear and tear of time.

Incorporating fasting into your daily routine doesn't have to be daunting. Start with a sustainable approach, choosing a fasting schedule that aligns with your lifestyle. Many find success with the 16:8 method. This routine offers flexibility, making it easier to adhere to while still reaping the longevity benefits. Consistency is key; even small, regular fasting periods can significantly improve health over time. Consider starting your fast after an early dinner and breaking it with a nutritious breakfast later in the morning, setting a rhythm that respects your body's natural cycles.

Expert insights provide further assurance of fasting's potential. Renowned gerontologists and nutritionists emphasize the role of fasting in promoting longevity. Dr. David Jockers, a doctor of natural medicine, highlights how fasting can downregulate nutrient-sensing pathways like mTOR, a cellular mechanism associated with growth and aging.[2] By modifying these pathways, fasting encourages the body to prioritize maintenance and repair rather than growth, enhancing health. An article from *Medical News Today* highlights that fasting may also help reduce inflammation in the body, noting that high-calorie diets are associated with chronic metabolic inflammatory syndromes.[3]

Interactive Element: Longevity Reflection Journal: To enhance

---

2. David Jockers, MD, "The Truth About mTOR, Autophagy and Longevity," the Dr. Jockers website, https://www.lifespan.io/news/intermittent-fasting-induces-changes-in-multiple-biomarkers.https://drjockers.com/episode-467-the-truth-about-mtor-autophagy-and-longevity/?utm_source=chatgpt.co.
3. Tony Hicks, "How fasting can reduce disease risk by lowering inflammation," February 2, 2024, Medical News Today, https://www.medicalnewstoday.com/articles/how-fasting-can-reduce-disease-risk-by-lowering-inflammation?utm_source=chatgpt.com.

your fasting practice and reflect on its benefits, consider keeping a longevity reflection journal. Use it to note any changes you observe in your energy levels, mood, or overall well-being as you incorporate fasting. Reflect on questions like:

- How has fasting influenced your daily routine and energy levels?
- Have you noticed any changes in your mood or mental clarity?
- What long-term health goals do you hope to achieve through fasting?

This journaling exercise can help you stay connected to your health journey, providing insights and motivation as you embrace fasting's potential to help you live longer.

AUTOPHAGY: CELLULAR RENEWAL THROUGH FASTING

Imagine your body as a bustling city, where each cell is a building and, over time, some buildings become run-down or damaged. Autophagy, a natural process in your body, acts like a cleanup crew, diligently removing and recycling these damaged components, much like workers renovating old structures to keep the city thriving.

This cellular renewal is essential for maintaining optimal health. Fasting has been shown to enhance autophagy, making it a valuable practice if you're seeking to improve your well-being as you age. By temporarily abstaining from food, you trigger a state in which your body prioritizes repair and maintenance, focusing on cellular housekeeping rather than growth. This shift supports cell health and plays a significant role in preventing diseases and mitigating the effects of aging.

One of the remarkable benefits of autophagy is its potential to reduce cancer risk. When cells are damaged or dysfunctional, they can sometimes become cancerous. Autophagy helps prevent this transformation by clearing out damaged cellular components before they become problematic. This process acts as a safeguard, reducing the risk of cells going rogue and turning into cancerous growths. By promoting cellular repair and integrity, autophagy supports a healthier internal environment, which is crucial for disease prevention. Additionally, autophagy has been linked to improved immune function, as it helps clear out pathogens and supports your body's defense mechanisms. This enhanced immune response further contributes to your ability to ward off illnesses and maintain overall health.

To maximize the benefits of autophagy through fasting, consider incorporating extended fasting periods into your routine. While daily fasting, such as the 16:8 method, is beneficial, longer fasting sessions can amplify autophagy. Extended fasting periods, ranging from twenty-four to forty-eight hours, offer your body a more substantial opportunity to engage in cellular cleanup. During these longer fasts, the absence of external energy sources prompts your body to rely on its internal resources, intensifying the autophagic process.

It's important to approach extended fasting with caution. Listen to your body and consult healthcare professionals if needed. Gradually building up to longer fasts can help you acclimate without overwhelming your system. Incorporating these fasting strategies into your lifestyle can foster a deeper level of cellular renewal, supporting long-term health and wellness.

Visual aids can be incredibly helpful in understanding the complex concept of autophagy. This diagram illustrates the process of breaking down a cell with damaged components and recycling it into new, healthy parts. It simplifies the intricate biological processes, making it easier to grasp how fasting influences cellular health.

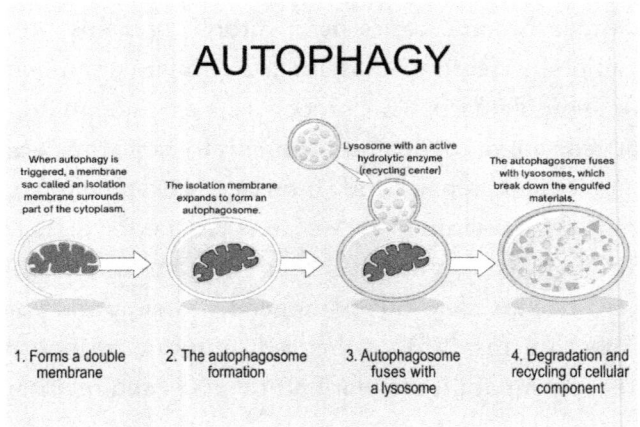

The goal here is to demystify the science behind autophagy and offer a clear, engaging way to visualize how fasting benefits cellular renewal. By understanding these processes, you can appreciate the profound impact fasting has on your body and motivate yourself to integrate it into your health regimen.

HEART HEALTH: FASTING'S IMPACT ON CARDIOVASCULAR WELLNESS

Your heart's health is foundational, and intermittent fasting has emerged as a powerful ally in maintaining cardiovascular wellness. One of the standout benefits of fasting is its ability to lower LDL cholesterol levels. LDL, often dubbed bad cholesterol, can accumulate in the arteries, leading to blockages and increasing the risk of heart disease. Fasting helps your body use its stored energy, lowering cholesterol levels and promoting a healthier heart. This process cleanses the bloodstream and helps the heart function more efficiently, providing a strong foundation for overall cardiovascular health.

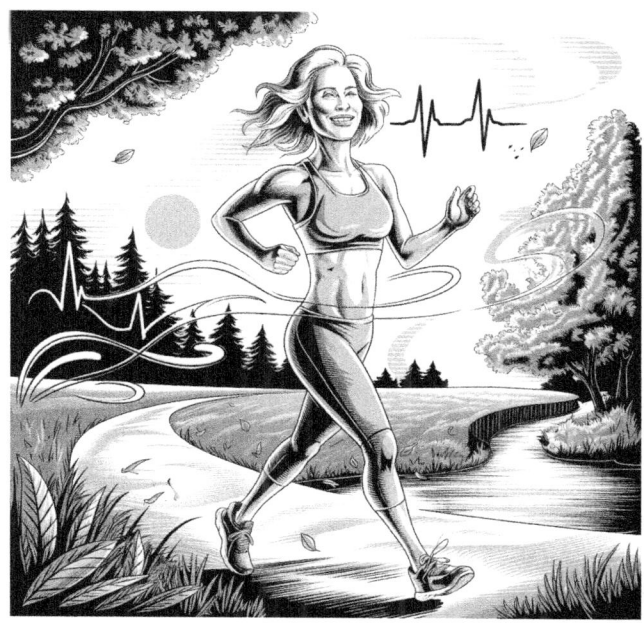

Fasting also plays a crucial role in regulating blood pressure. High blood pressure forces the heart to work harder than necessary, which increases the risk of heart attacks and strokes. Fasting has been shown to improve vascular function, allowing blood to flow more freely through the arteries and reducing the strain on the heart. This improvement in blood pressure is pivotal in mitigating the risks associated with heart disease because it fosters a more resilient cardiovascular system. Fasting's impact on heart health is further supported by evidence showing that regular fasting can lower the incidence of heart-related issues and offers a proactive approach to maintaining a healthy heart as we age.[4]

While fasting lays a robust groundwork for cardiovascular health, it's most effective when combined with other heart-healthy

---

4. Kat Long, "Intermittent fasting may protect the heart by controlling inflammation," November 18, 2021, The American Heart Association website, https://www.heart.org/en/news/2021/11/18/intermittent-fasting-may-protect-the-heart-by-controlling-inflammation?utm_source=chatgpt.com.

habits. Stress management, for instance, is a key component of heart care. High stress levels can lead to increased blood pressure and a higher heart rate, which strain the cardiovascular system. Incorporating yoga, breathwork, and meditation can significantly reduce stress, promoting a calm and balanced state of mind. These practices soothe the soul and directly benefit the heart by lowering stress-induced physiological responses.

Regular physical activity, such as brisk walking or cycling, is another essential habit that complements fasting. Exercise strengthens the heart muscle, improves circulation, and enhances overall cardiovascular fitness, creating a holistic approach to heart health.

> **Maureen's Story:** Take Maureen. In her mid-fifties, she found herself facing high cholesterol and blood pressure. Although she tried various diets and medications, the results were not as promising as she had hoped. It was only after adopting intermittent fasting, along with yoga and mindful eating and breathing, that she noticed significant improvements. Her LDL cholesterol dropped, and her blood pressure stabilized, allowing her to reduce her reliance on medication.

Stories like Maureen's highlight the real-world benefits of fasting for heart health. Many women have shared similar stories, reporting improved cardiovascular markers and a renewed stamina and confidence. These accounts reinforce the idea that fasting, coupled with intentional lifestyle changes, can create a positive ripple effect throughout the body. By choosing to focus on heart health, you're investing in the physical aspects and enhancing your overall quality of life. It's a journey that offers both immediate and long-term rewards, empowering you to take control of your heart health with confidence and care.

REDUCING DIABETES RISK WITH FASTING PRACTICES

Maintaining balanced blood sugar levels can sometimes feel like a complex choreography in the dance of life. As we age, our bodies might not respond to insulin as efficiently as they once did. This condition, known as insulin resistance, is a precursor to type 2 diabetes. Insulin helps cells absorb glucose (sugar) from the bloodstream for energy. When cells resist insulin, glucose builds up in the blood, leading to high blood sugar levels.

This is where intermittent fasting steps onto the stage, offering a promising role in improving insulin sensitivity. Giving your body regular breaks from food allows insulin levels to drop, encouraging cells to become more responsive to insulin when you eat. This process can enhance glucose metabolism, making it an effective strategy for lowering diabetes risk.

Intermittent fasting is like a well-orchestrated routine, with various styles to suit different preferences. If you're aiming to reduce your risk of diabetes, specific fasting protocols can be particularly beneficial. The 16:8 method helps regulate blood sugar levels, giving your body consistent periods to reset and improve insulin function. You might also consider alternate-day fasting, in which you alternate between regular eating days and days with reduced calorie intake. Each of these methods offers a structured way to help your body manage blood sugar levels more effectively, potentially preventing the onset of diabetes.

Complementing fasting with a diet focused on regulating blood sugar can further enhance its benefits. Opt for foods with a low glycemic index (GI), which means they have a slower, more gradual impact on blood sugar levels. Berries, for instance, are an excellent choice. They're delicious, packed with antioxidants, and have a low GI. Nuts, another wise option, provide healthy fats and protein, helping stabilize blood sugar. Whole grains, legumes, and vegetables, like leafy greens, should also feature prominently in your meals. By choosing these foods, you support your body's natural ability to manage blood sugar and create a harmonious balance that aligns with your fasting practices.

While fasting can be a powerful tool for preventing diabetes, it's crucial to proceed with care. If you have diabetes or pre-diabetes, consult with your healthcare providers before starting a fasting regimen. Medical supervision ensures that fasting is safe and suitable for your individual circumstances. Your healthcare provider can help tailor a fasting plan that considers your current health status and any medications you're taking. This personalized approach is key to reaping the benefits of fasting while minimizing potential risks. It's essential to regularly monitor blood sugar levels, especially if you're on insulin or other diabetes medications, to avoid hypoglycemia (low blood sugar) or other complications.

Fasting, combined with a mindful diet and medical guidance, becomes a formidable ally in reducing diabetes risk. By adopting these practices, you support your body's natural insulin function and embrace a lifestyle that promotes overall health.

ENHANCING DIGESTIVE HEALTH AND GUT BALANCE

Imagine your gut as the bustling center of your body's ecosystem, teeming with trillions of microorganisms that play a crucial role in your overall health. These tiny inhabitants, collectively known as the microbiome, are fundamental for digestion, immunity, and mood regulation. Fasting offers a unique opportunity to support this delicate balance, promoting a diverse and healthy microbiome. When you fast, your digestive system gets a much-needed rest, allowing your gut flora to flourish. This period of rest can increase microbiome diversity, which is essential for a resilient digestive system. A diverse microbiome is like having a robust library of resources at your body's disposal, ready to tackle challenges and maintain health.

One of the most immediate benefits of fasting is that it reduces bloating. We've all experienced that uncomfortable, swollen feeling after a heavy meal or a particularly stressful day. Fasting gives your digestive tract time to reset, reducing the buildup of gases and allowing your intestines to calm. This can noticeably decrease bloating, leaving you feeling lighter and more comfortable. Additionally, the rest period helps make your digestion more efficient, enhancing your ability to absorb nutrients and eliminate waste. With less constant demand for digestion, your gut can repair and optimize its functions, making your digestive process more regular and comfortable.

To maximize the digestive benefits of fasting, consider incorporating alternate-day fasting into your routine. It involves fasting every other day, allowing your digestive system ample time to recover and heal. It also balances the need for nourishment with the advantages of digestive rest. On fasting days, focus on staying hydrated, as water helps flush out toxins and supports cellular processes. On eating days, prioritize foods that nourish and support gut health. Fermented foods, like yogurt and kimchi, are fantastic additions to your diet. Rich in probiotics, these foods introduce beneficial bacteria, enhancing your gut's health and diversity. Yogurt, with its creamy texture and tangy flavor, offers a delicious way to support your gut. Meanwhile, kimchi, a spicy fermented cabbage, adds a kick to meals and boosts gut flora.

A sample meal plan:

- **Breakfast:** Yogurt topped with berries and a sprinkle of chia seeds. This meal is gut-friendly and packed with antioxidants and fiber.
- **Lunch:** A quinoa salad with a generous helping of mixed greens, cherry tomatoes, and a dollop of kimchi. The combination of fiber and probiotics supports digestion and satisfies hunger.
- **Dinner:** A lean protein, like grilled chicken or tofu, paired with fermented vegetables and a side of roasted sweet potatoes.

These meals are designed to be easy on the digestive system while offering the nutrients necessary for energy and health.

FASTING AS A TOOL FOR DISEASE PREVENTION

Intermittent fasting offers a powerful strategy for reducing the risk of chronic diseases by focusing on prevention through healthy cellular function. Fasting helps prevent disease by reducing cell proliferation, a critical factor in cancer development. By limiting the constant influx of nutrients, fasting slows down the pace at which cells divide and grow. This slowdown provides a critical checkpoint, reducing the chances of abnormal cells multiplying uncontrollably. In this way, fasting acts as a natural regulator, keeping cellular growth in check and lowering the risk of cancerous changes.

As mentioned earlier, fasting also shines in its ability to reduce inflammation, a known contributor to many chronic diseases. Inflammation, while a natural response to injury or infection, can become problematic when it persists unchecked, leading to conditions like arthritis, heart disease, and even Alzheimer's. Intermittent fasting helps control chronic inflammation by modulating the body's inflammatory response. When you fast, your body reduces the production of pro-inflammatory markers, creating a more balanced internal environment. This reduction in inflammation helps prevent disease and supports overall health, leaving you feeling more energetic. By incorporating fasting into your routine, you give your body regular opportunities to reset and heal, paving the way for a healthier future.

To maintain overall health and maximize the disease-preventing benefits of fasting, it's important to combine fasting with a balanced lifestyle. This means integrating fasting into a daily routine that includes nutritious meals and regular physical activity. Pair a fasting schedule that fits your lifestyle with a diet rich in whole foods. Incorporate a variety of vegetables, lean proteins, and healthy fats to ensure that you're getting the nutrients your body needs. Physical activity, even something as simple as daily walks, complements fasting by enhancing metabolic health and further reducing inflammation. By creating a routine that balances fasting with healthy living habits, you foster an environment where your body can thrive.

For those interested in delving deeper into the science and benefits of fasting, there's a wealth of resources available. *The Complete Guide to Fasting* by Dr. Jason Fung and *The Longevity Diet* by Valter Longo provide in-depth insights into how fasting supports health. Additionally, studies published in scientific journals offer a deeper understanding of fasting's impact on disease prevention, including from the *Journal of the Academy of Nutrition and Dietetics*.

It's clear that fasting offers more than just a strategy for weight management or energy regulation. Its potential for disease prevention is profound, providing a natural and effective approach to improving health. By embracing fasting as part of your routine, you empower yourself with a tool that supports your body's defenses against chronic diseases, paving the way for a future filled with health and well-being.

7
INTERACTIVE ELEMENTS AND PERSONALIZED FASTING JOURNEYS

"Your visions will become clear only when you can look into your own heart. Who looks outside, dreams; who looks inside, awakes." — Carl Jung

As women navigating the dynamic yet sometimes challenging phase of life over forty, we can capture our discoveries and reflections through journaling to transform this journey into a masterpiece of personal growth. Journaling isn't just about putting pen to paper. It's about creating a space to explore your thoughts, track your progress, and truly connect with your body and mind. This practice offers a way to reflect on how fasting affects you, providing insights that might otherwise go unnoticed.

Journaling during your fasting journey can be a powerful tool for enhancing self-awareness. It allows you to pause and consider the changes you've noticed in your energy levels and how your mood varies before and after fasting. These observations help reveal patterns, making it easier to identify what works best for you. For instance, you might discover that fasting on certain days boosts your energy and requires more rest on others.

Reflect on the following questions to understand your unique response to fasting:

- "What changes have I noticed in my energy levels?"
- "How do I feel before and after fasting?"

Structured journaling prompts can help you capture these reflections more effectively. Daily reflections are a great starting point, encouraging you to note both your physical and emotional states. You could jot down how your body feels, any noticeable shifts in mood, and even small victories like resisting a craving or trying a new healthy recipe.

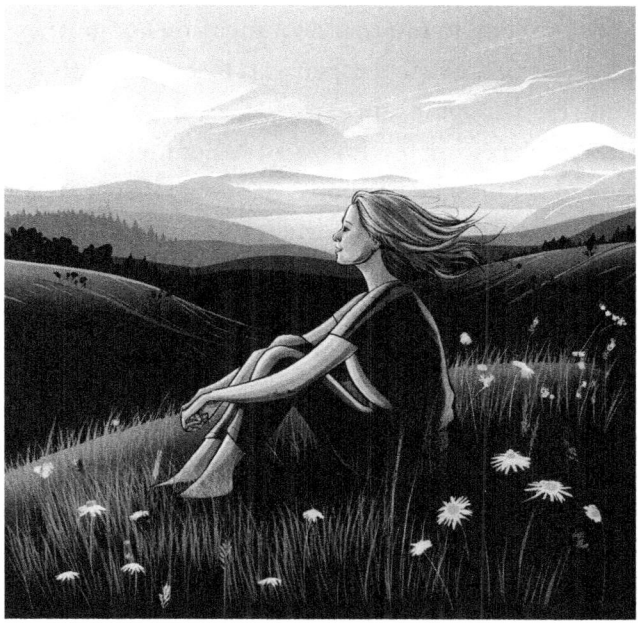

Weekly summaries take this a step further, allowing you to assess your progress and challenges over an extended period. This broader view helps you see trends and adjust your fasting routine. By regularly engaging with these prompts, you create a narrative of your fasting journey that highlights both achievements and areas for growth.

Journaling keeps you accountable. Writing down your experiences can remind you of your goals and motivations, reinforcing your commitment to intermittent fasting. It acts as a personal coach, gently nudging you to stay on track even when the going gets tough. Many women find that journaling helps them stay focused and motivated, especially during moments of doubt or temptation. The act of writing itself can be empowering, reaffirming your dedication to health and wellness every time you put pen to paper.

Sandy's Story: Sandy began journaling as part of her fasting practice. Initially, she wasn't sure if it would make a difference, but she soon found that documenting her journey provided clarity and encouragement. By consistently recording her thoughts and experiences, she was able to identify which fasting methods suited her lifestyle and which foods nourished her body. Her journal became a trusted companion, offering insights and inspiration whenever she needed it. Through daily entries, Sandy tracked patterns in her energy levels and mood, allowing her to fine-tune her fasting over time. This consistency helped her achieve her health goals and deepened her connection with herself.

Interactive Element: Journaling Prompts for Self-Discovery:
Explore your fasting experience with these journaling prompts:

1. **Daily reflections:** Note physical sensations, emotional shifts, and any notable experiences throughout your fasting and eating windows.
2. **Weekly summaries:** Assess your overall progress,

celebrating successes and recognizing challenges. Consider what adjustments might enhance your journey.
3. **Monthly review:** Look back over the month to spot patterns and trends. Reflect on what you've learned and how you might continue to grow.

By embracing journaling as part of your fasting journey, you open the door to greater self-awareness and empowerment. This practice supports your physical health and nurtures your emotional well-being, creating a holistic approach to wellness that honors every aspect of who you are.

DESIGNING YOUR PERSONALIZED FASTING PLAN

Creating a fasting plan that fits your life is like tailoring a dress—it must be suited to your unique shape and needs to be truly comfortable.

Start by defining your health objectives. What do you hope to achieve through intermittent fasting? Whether it's shedding a few pounds, balancing hormones, or boosting your energy levels, having clear goals will guide your choices. Once these goals are set, consider how fasting can fit into your lifestyle. Are you an early bird or a night owl? Your natural rhythm will help determine the best fasting windows for you. Maybe you prefer the 16:8 method, which allows you to eat within an eight-hour window. Or perhaps a more flexible approach suits you better, like the 5:2 method, in which you eat normally for five days and restrict calories for two.

To help bring your plan to life, use tools like printable templates (free downloadable templates are available with this book) or create your own. These are a visual guide for scheduling your eating and fasting periods, making it easier to stick to your plan. Templates allow for flexibility, encouraging you to adjust fasting windows as your needs change. Perhaps you find that fasting from seven p.m. to eleven a.m. works well during the week, but you need different hours on weekends. Customize your schedule to fit your life. And don't be afraid to make changes as you learn what works best.

It's important to revisit and revise your fasting plan regularly. Just like health goals evolve, so do lifestyles and needs. What worked for you last month might need tweaking today. Set aside time every few weeks to evaluate your fasting strategy. Are you meeting your goals? Do you feel energized and balanced? If not, consider what adjustments might help. It could be as simple as shifting your fasting window or incorporating new foods that better support your energy levels. This ongoing refinement ensures that your plan remains effective and aligned with your well-being.

> **Julie's Story:** Julie struggled at first to find a fasting routine that fit her life. She tried the 16:8 method but realized it clashed with her busy mornings. So she switched to the 14:10 method, which allowed her to enjoy early workouts and family breakfasts without stress. Her journey shows how important it is to stay flexible and find what works for you. Everyone's body and daily routine are unique, so don't be afraid to adjust and make fasting fit your lifestyle.

> **Janet's Story:** Janet wanted to focus on weight loss and mental clarity. She began with the 5:2 method, which allowed her to enjoy social meals without restriction on most days. By incorporating mindfulness practices and nutrient-dense foods on her fasting days, she experienced improved focus and gradual weight loss. Her personalized plan became a sustainable part of her lifestyle, demonstrating that fasting can be both enjoyable and effective.

Interactive Element: Personalized Fasting Plan Template: Use this template to design your custom fasting plan:

- **Fasting goals:** Define what you want to achieve with fasting (weight, sleep, mindful eating).
- **Preferred methods:** Choose your fasting approach (e.g., 16:8, 5:2) and adjust as needed.
- **Fasting schedule:** Outline your daily or weekly fasting windows.
- **Exercise type and duration:** Outline your preferred daily exercise and time/length of activities.
- **Hydration Strategy:** Water intake during fasting window and Beverages allowed during eating window.
- **Review and adjust:** Revisit and revise your strategy every few weeks.

IF FASTING PLAN
Customize Your Own Personalized Approach

Fasting Goals
Define what you want to achieve:

Preferred Methods
Choose your fasting approach (e.g., 16:8, 14:10, 5:2):

Fasting Schedule
Monday-Sunday - Fast Hours;
Eating Hours:

Exercise Type & Duration
Outline your preferred daily exercise and time/length of activities:

Support Tools to Be Used

Apps:

Community groups:

Journaling approach:

Meal planning approach:

Hydration Strategy

Review Strategy
Revisit and revise your strategy

By personalizing your fasting plan, you create a path that supports your unique journey toward better health. Enjoy the flexibility to adapt, knowing that the plan is there to serve you, not the other way around.

TRACKING TOOLS FOR FASTING SUCCESS

Imagine starting your day with a clear plan, knowing exactly when your fasting window begins and ends. Tracking your progress in intermittent fasting can be a game-changer, providing you with insights that go beyond mere numbers. It's not just about meeting goals but understanding your body better. Keeping a record of when you fast, how you feel, and what you eat can highlight patterns and reveal what works for you.

Digital fasting apps have become an invaluable resource, offering an easy way to log fasting windows and track your progress. Apps like Zero, Simple, and FastHabit help you keep track and provide reminders, ensuring that you stay consistent. These tools are designed to fit seamlessly into your life, making it easier to stick with your fasting routine and adjust as needed.

If you prefer a more tactile approach, fasting journals offer a hands-on way to monitor your journey. Writing down your daily fasting schedule and how you feel during eating and fasting periods can create a tangible connection to your progress. These journals can be as simple or detailed as you like. Some women jot down quick notes in a notebook, while others use structured templates that guide them in capturing more detailed information. The act of manually recording your experiences can be therapeutic, offering a moment of reflection in a busy day. It allows you to see the big picture and make informed decisions about any changes needed in your fasting strategy.

INTERMITTENT FASTING JOURNAL

Date: ___ / ___ / ___ **Fasting Day:** ○ Yes ○ No

Sleep
- To Bed ___
- Wake Up ___
- Hours Slept ___
- Quality ___

- First Bite ___
- Last Bite ___
- Fasting Hours ___
- Eating Hours ___

My Daily Goals

My Motivation

Exercise Type ___ **Duration** ___

Meals and Snacks
○ Breakfast ○ Lunch ○ Dinner ○ Snacks

- ___ Calories: ___
- ___ Calories: ___
- ___ Calories: ___
- ___ Calories: ___
- ___ Calories: ___
- ___ Calories: ___

Water Intake

Energy Level

Feel

Notes ___

Apps provide features that can make tracking even more insightful. Many let you log not just fasting windows but also food intake, water consumption, and exercise. Some even integrate with wearables for a comprehensive view of your health. This data can be incredibly useful when you're trying to correlate fasting with energy levels or mood changes. Perhaps you'll notice that on days when you break your fast with a protein-rich meal, your energy remains stable throughout the day. Or maybe you'll find that shortening your fasting window or aligning your eating window with peak energy times on stressful days helps you stay focused and calm.

Using tracking data effectively involves more than just collecting information. It's about interpreting what it means for you. Look for patterns that emerge over time. Do you have more energy on days when you fast for a certain number of hours? Are there particular foods that leave you feeling sluggish or energized? By identifying these patterns, you can tailor your fasting and eating habits to align with your body's needs. This personalization is key to making fasting a sustainable and successful part of your lifestyle. It's like having a map that guides you toward better health, one data point at a time.

Consistency in tracking is crucial for gaining meaningful insights. Setting reminders can help make tracking a regular part of your routine. Most apps allow you to set alerts to log your fasting start and end times so you don't forget. If you use a paper journal, placing it somewhere you'll see it every day, like on your nightstand or next to your morning coffee, can serve as a gentle prompt. The goal is to make tracking a habit—something you do without thinking, much like brushing your teeth. This consistency helps you stay on track with your fasting goals and builds a rich repository of data that can inform and inspire your fasting journey.

Incorporating these tracking tools into your intermittent fasting practice can significantly enhance your understanding and control over your health. Whether you choose apps or a more traditional journal, the key is finding a method that resonates with you and complements your lifestyle. With the right tools and a bit of dedication, you can get a deeper insight into how fasting affects your body and make informed decisions that support your well-being.

SUCCESS STORIES: REAL-LIFE TRANSFORMATIONS

Like many women, Katie found herself battling persistent weight gain in her late forties. Even though she tried various diets, nothing seemed to work until she embraced intermittent fasting. By adopting a 16:8 fasting schedule, Katie gradually lost twenty pounds over several months. But it was more than the number on the scale. The return of her energy and confidence marked her success. She found herself participating in activities she once loved but had set aside, like hiking and dancing. Katie's story isn't just about weight loss. It's about rediscovering joy and a zest for life—something that resonates deeply with many of us.

Then there's Michelle, who struggled with debilitating hot flashes and mood swings during menopause. They affected her work, relationships, and overall quality of life. After researching various options, she decided to try intermittent fasting, intrigued by its potential to balance hormones. Within a few weeks, she noticed significantly fewer symptoms. Her flashes became less frequent and less intense, and her mood stabilized. Michelle also welcomed the emotional lift that came with it. She felt more in control and more herself, and this transformation extended beyond her personal life into her professional world, where she felt more focused and confident.

What makes these stories compelling is not just the end result but the journey—the emotional highs and lows, the perseverance through challenges, and the celebration of small victories along the way. These elements bring depth and relatability, making it easy to see ourselves in these women's shoes. Success stories often begin with a struggle and the realization that something needs to change. The women evolve through experimentation and adaptation as they find what works for them. These narratives are filled with resilience, a willingness to try, fail, and try again. They inspire us to push through our own challenges, knowing that others have faced similar obstacles and emerged stronger.

As you embark on your own fasting adventure, consider documenting your experiences. Your story is powerful, and it deserves to be told. Start by tracking your progress, noting not just the physical changes but the emotional shifts as well. Capture the essence of your growth by reflecting on your challenges and successes. Think about what motivates you and how fasting has influenced your life.

This isn't just about numbers or metrics but the journey toward a healthier, more thriving you. Sharing your story can serve as an inspiration to others and a reminder of how far you've come. Just like Katie and Michelle, your experiences can become a beacon of hope and encouragement, illustrating the transformative power of intermittent fasting.

COMMUNITY AND SUPPORT: BUILDING CONNECTIONS

Finding a community can be a lifeline when embarking on the intermittent fasting journey, especially when you hit those inevitable bumps along the road. Connecting with others who understand the unique challenges of fasting can offer both motivation and support. Imagine having a group that cheers you on during your successes and lifts you up during challenges. This sense of belonging can make all the difference.

Online forums have become welcoming spaces where people share their experiences, seek advice, and find camaraderie. These platforms allow you to tap into a wealth of collective wisdom, offering tips and encouragement that can help you stay on track. Whether it's a simple question about fasting windows or a deeper discussion about personal struggles, these forums provide a supportive environment where you can learn and grow alongside others.

Social media groups are another fantastic avenue for finding fasting-focused communities. Facebook and Reddit host numerous groups dedicated to intermittent fasting, where you can connect with individuals who share your interests and goals. These groups often host discussions, share success stories, and provide a space for members to ask questions and offer insights. Engaging in these communities can help you feel less isolated, knowing that others are navigating similar paths.

In-person gatherings, such as local meetups or fasting circles, offer a more personal connection. Meeting face-to-face with others who are also on their fasting journey can create powerful bonds. These gatherings often include group discussions, shared meals, and opportunities to learn from guest speakers or experienced fasters. The shared experience of fasting can foster unity and provide a network of support that extends beyond the digital realm.

Sharing your experiences with others reinforces your commitment and offers a chance to learn from different perspectives. Discussing challenges and successes with others can provide encouragement and spark new ideas. You might discover tips for overcoming cravings or learn about new recipes that fit your fasting plan. Hearing about others' experiences can also remind you that you're not alone in your struggles and that you can achieve success with persistence and support.

> **Anne's Story:** Consider Anne, who joined a local fasting group in her community. Initially hesitant, she found that the shared experience of fasting created a deep bond with other members. They met weekly to discuss their progress, exchange recipes, and provide mutual support. The group's accountability helped Anne stay on track, and she cherished the friendships that blossomed from their shared journey.

Peer support systems can play a crucial role in building accountability partnerships. Having someone to check in with regularly can motivate you to stay committed to your fasting goals. This could be a friend, family member, or someone you've met through a fasting community. Regular check-ins, whether through phone calls, messages, or in-person meetings, provide a space to share updates, celebrate victories, and tackle challenges together. Accountability partnerships create shared responsibility, helping both parties remain focused and motivated.

>**Jane and Lisa's Story:** They met in an online fasting forum and quickly realized they had similar goals and challenges. The two decided to become accountability partners, checking in with each other daily. This partnership provided the encouragement they needed to stay committed, and they celebrated each other's milestones along the way. Their connection grew beyond fasting, becoming a friendship that enriched their lives in many ways.

ENCOURAGING ADAPTABILITY AND OPEN-MINDEDNESS

In the world of intermittent fasting, adaptability is a key skill. Life rarely stays the same, and as we age, our schedules, responsibilities, and even our bodies change. Embracing flexibility in your fasting routine can make the difference between a short-lived experiment and a lasting lifestyle change. Imagine, for instance, a week in which work demands suddenly increase or family obligations shift, making your usual fasting window impractical. Instead of abandoning your efforts, adaptability allows you to adjust. Perhaps you shift your fasting hours or choose a different fasting method altogether. This flexibility ensures that fasting remains a supportive practice rather than a rigid rule. Recently, I was on a family vacation that took me to a different time zone. It became challenging to stick to my fasting schedule. Rather than getting frustrated, I went with the flow and did my best to adjust my schedule and get back on track.

Being open-minded is equally important. When you approach fasting with curiosity and a willingness to explore, you allow yourself to discover what truly works for you. New experiences can bring about unexpected insights, enriching your fasting practice. Maybe you try a new fasting method, like the crescendo method, which involves fasting for shorter periods on nonconsecutive days. By staying open to new possibilities, you give yourself the chance to grow and learn. This openness applies to fasting hours, new foods, exercise routines, and mindfulness practices that complement your fasting.

Resistance to change is natural, but growth happens when you overcome it. If the idea of altering your routine feels daunting, start small. Incremental adjustments can make significant changes more manageable. For example, if you're used to fasting for twelve hours, try extending it by thirty minutes. See how your body responds before deciding on further changes. These small shifts build confidence and make larger transitions feel less overwhelming. Also, consider setting small goals that align with these changes. As you achieve each one, you'll gain momentum and motivation to continue adapting.

When it comes to fostering adaptability, mindset plays a crucial role. Viewing challenges as opportunities for growth can transform how you approach difficulties. Instead of seeing a disrupted fasting window as a setback, see it as a chance to try something new. Maybe it's an opportunity to experiment with a different fasting schedule or focus on nutrition during your eating window. By shifting your mindset, you can turn obstacles into stepping stones, each one leading you closer to your goals. This positive outlook enhances your fasting practice and spills over into other areas of life, creating a more resilient and adaptable you.

To encourage adaptability, remind yourself of the bigger picture. What are your ultimate health goals? How does fasting help you achieve them? Keeping these in mind can motivate you to remain flexible and open to change.

Remember, intermittent fasting is not about perfection. It's about progress. Each adjustment you make, each new method you try, brings you closer to understanding what works best for you.

Celebrate these small victories, as they are the building blocks of lasting success. With an adaptable approach, you'll find that fasting becomes a seamless part of your life—one that supports your health and well-being through every twist and turn.

8

INTEGRATING FASTING INTO EVERYDAY LIFE

"The passion for stretching yourself and sticking to it, even when it's not going well, is the hallmark of the growth mindset." — Carol Dweck

Successfully integrating intermittent fasting into your daily routine requires thoughtful planning and a gradual approach that respects your lifestyle and commitments. Rather than diving into an ambitious fasting schedule immediately, start by pushing your breakfast back by an hour every few days until you reach your desired fasting window. This gentle transition allows your body to adapt while minimizing discomfort and the likelihood that you'll give up. Pay special attention to your work schedule, social commitments, and exercise routine when choosing your eating window. For instance, if you typically have business lunches or family dinners, ensure that your eating window accommodates these important meals. Similarly, if you exercise in the morning, you might want to schedule your eating window to begin shortly after your workout to support recovery.

For many women over forty, maintaining healthy habits like intermittent fasting while balancing family and a social life can feel like juggling too many balls. The key to managing this is open communication and strategic planning. When you choose to embrace fasting, it's important to share your goals and the reasons behind them with your family. This helps set clear expectations and opens up a channel for support and understanding. Explain the health benefits you've discovered and how fasting contributes to your overall well-being. Family meetings can be a great way to lay everything on the table, literally and figuratively. Discuss your fasting schedule and how it might affect meal times or social activities. This proactive approach allows your loved ones to align with your needs, making the transition smoother for everyone.

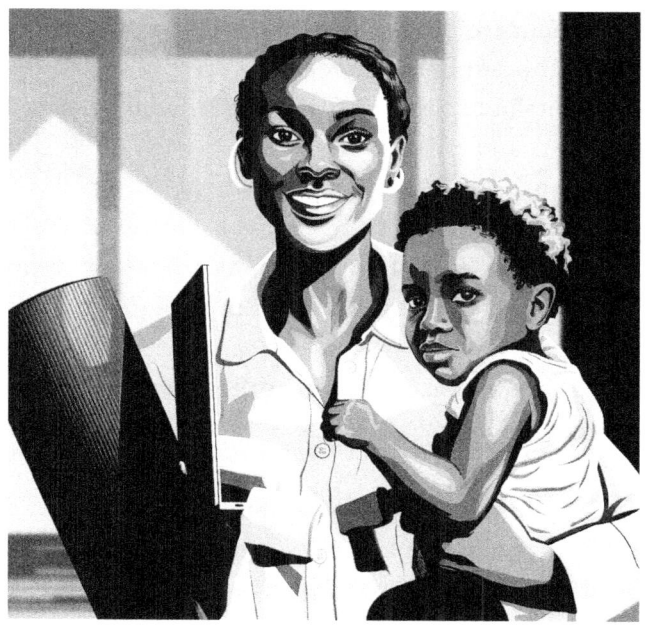

Meal planning becomes an essential tool in harmonizing fasting with family dynamics. Since a household can have diverse dietary needs, finding recipes that can cater to everyone might seem daunting. However, it can also be an opportunity to get creative in the kitchen. Consider meals that are easy to adapt, like a hearty vegetable soup that can be enriched with different proteins or grains, depending on individual preferences.

Batch cooking can also help. In my case, I have a family of five and work full-time. So making things easier is essential. When you prepare meals in advance, you save time on busy days and ensure that nutritious, fasting-friendly options are always within reach. This strategy supports your fasting goals and provides peace of mind since you know that you have healthy meals ready to go. It also reduces the temptation to stray from your plan.

Involving your family in the fasting journey can transform it from an individual pursuit into a shared experience. Cooking together can serve as a bonding activity in which everyone learns about the benefits of the nutritious ingredients you choose to include. Share the responsibility of meal prep, allowing each family member to contribute to the process. This lightens your load and fosters teamwork and inclusion.

Social dining, a staple in many households, can pose challenges. But with a little foresight, it can be enjoyable and stress-free. When dining out, suggest restaurants with menus that offer flexible options, making it easier to find dishes that align with your fasting schedule. Look for places that serve a variety of salads, grilled proteins, or vegetable-based dishes, as these tend to be more adaptable to different dietary needs.

Interactive Element: Family Meal-Planning Guide: Gather your family together for a meal-planning session. Use this guide to brainstorm fasting-friendly recipes and plan out the week's meals:

- **Family favorites:** List everyone's favorite dishes and identify those that can be easily modified to fit fasting needs.
- **Batch cooking day:** Choose one day a week when everyone helps prepare meals in bulk. Assign tasks to each person to make the process efficient.

- **Restaurant night:** Select one night to dine out. Research menus in advance to ensure that options are suitable for your fasting plan.

By incorporating these strategies, you create a supportive environment in which fasting becomes a natural part of your everyday life. This integration benefits your health and enriches your relationships as you share in the journey together.

FASTING AT WORK: TIPS FOR BUSY PROFESSIONALS

If you are like me, a typical workday includes back-to-back meetings, looming deadlines, and the constant buzz of office life. Now, add intermittent fasting into the mix.

It might seem daunting, but fasting can be seamlessly integrated into even the busiest professional setting with the right strategies. The key is preparation, and it starts before you even set foot in the office. Meal prepping for workdays is a lifesaver. When you prepare in advance lunches that align with your fasting schedule, you won't be caught off guard by hunger or tempted by the less healthy options that might lurk in the break room. A simple, satisfying salad with lean proteins and a variety of fresh vegetables can be a go-to. Throw in some nuts or seeds for a crunch and healthy fats, and you've got a meal that supports your fasting goals and keeps you energized through the afternoon slump.

Once at work, how you use your breaks can make a significant difference in maintaining your fasting routine. Instead of reaching for a snack, consider using that time to take a short walk or meditate. Both activities help clear your mind and reset your focus, enhancing productivity. A brisk walk outside can refresh your perspective, while a few minutes of meditation at your desk can calm the mind and reduce stress. By purposefully using your breaks, you support both your fasting practice and your work performance, creating a balance that benefits both areas of your life.

The benefits of fasting at work extend beyond physical health. They also enhance mental clarity and focus. Many people notice that they can concentrate better during fasting periods, experiencing a sharper mind and increased alertness. You can harness this clarity to tackle challenging tasks or creative projects. By scheduling demanding work during your fasting window, you might find yourself more productive and efficient, completing tasks with ease and precision. It's a subtle shift that can lead to significant improvements in your work performance and satisfaction.

However, navigating fasting in a workplace requires some finesse, especially when it comes to communicating your needs. It's important to address fasting with colleagues in a polite and clear way. If office lunches are a regular occurrence, consider suggesting alternatives or politely declining. You might say something like, "I'm following a specific eating schedule, but I'd love to join for coffee afterward." This approach includes you in social interactions without compromising your fasting goals. It's all about finding a balance that respects both your health choices and your professional relationships.

Time management is another critical aspect of balancing work responsibilities with fasting. Prioritizing tasks can help you use energy efficiently, especially during fasting periods. Start your day with a clear plan, focusing on high-priority tasks when your concentration is at its peak. Break tasks into smaller, manageable chunks, then allocate time for each. This method makes you more productive and prevents burnout, allowing you to maintain energy throughout the day. By organizing your tasks effectively, you can get a lot done and stay aligned with your fasting goals.

Integrating fasting into your work life is about creating harmony between your professional and personal health goals. It's about finding the strategies that work best for you and adapting them to your unique circumstances. When you're prepared, mindful, and clear, you can make fasting a natural part of your work routine, enhancing both your health and your productivity.

HANDLING SOCIAL EVENTS AND TRAVEL WHILE FASTING

Navigating social events while maintaining your fasting routine can initially seem like a high-wire act. However, with a bit of planning, it becomes more manageable. Start by checking the event menu ahead of time. Knowing what they offer beforehand lets you make informed decisions that align with your fasting goals. If you're attending a dinner, it might be helpful to schedule your eating window to coincide with the event. This way, you can enjoy your meal without breaking your fasting schedule.

Is it a potluck? You could bring a dish that suits your dietary needs so there's at least one option that supports your fasting. I've even eaten a small meal before going to an event to make sure I'm getting the micronutrients that align with my daily fasting plans.

Traveling adds another layer of complexity to fasting, yet it can also be an opportunity to practice flexibility. Packing your own snacks can be a game-changer. Opt for nonperishable, healthy options like nuts, dried fruit, or protein bars. These are convenient and help you avoid the unhealthy temptations that come with travel. Adjusting your fasting windows to accommodate different time zones can also ease the transition. If you're flying halfway across the globe, consider shifting your fasting schedule gradually in the days leading up to your trip. This helps your body adjust to a new time zone and maintains the rhythm you've worked hard to establish.

The magic word here is *flexibility*. While it's important to stay committed to your fasting goals, it's equally important to allow occasional adjustments, especially during travel or social gatherings. Life is full of unexpected events, and sometimes, it's okay to veer off the path slightly. This adaptability can prevent you from feeling restricted or deprived, making fasting a sustainable lifestyle choice. If you adjust your fasting window or indulge a bit more than usual, don't see it as a setback. Instead, view it as a conscious choice that enhances your overall experience. Balance is key, and flexibility is your friend.

Staying committed to your fasting routine amid the chaos of travel and social events is no small feat, but with intentionality, it becomes second nature. One strategy is mindful indulgence. This doesn't mean abandoning your fasting principles but rather enjoying special occasions without guilt. The holidays are a challenge for me, so I'm a little easier on myself and allow myself flexibility during this time. Choose indulgences that bring you joy, then savor them. This mindful approach allows you to enjoy the moment while maintaining control over your eating habits. You might find that when you focus on the quality rather than the quantity of indulgence, you can fully participate in social settings without feeling like you've compromised your fasting goals.

EMBRACING FASTING AS A LIFELONG HEALTH STRATEGY

Waking up each morning feeling empowered, knowing that the choices you make today contribute to your long-term well-being, is empowering. This is the essence of adopting intermittent fasting as a sustainable lifestyle choice. For many women over forty, the prospect of integrating fasting into daily life might seem daunting at first. Yet the long-term benefits of this practice can be profound and life-enhancing. Intermittent fasting is not just about skipping meals. It's about committing to a path of wellness that evolves with you. It offers lifelong improvements by supporting metabolic health, aiding in weight management, and enhancing mental clarity. As you continue to embrace fasting, these benefits accumulate, providing a foundation for sustained health and resilience.

Adapting fasting practices over time is crucial as your body and life change. What works perfectly in one stage may need tweaking in another. Aging shifts nutritional needs and energy levels, and fasting should reflect these transitions. In your forties, you might find that a

16:8 schedule suits your rhythm, but as you move into your fifties or sixties, you may prefer shorter fasting windows or different patterns, like 5:2. Your fasting plan should grow and adapt as you do, reflecting changes in lifestyle, activity levels, and health goals. This flexibility ensures that fasting remains an effective tool for health management, tailored to meet your evolving needs.

Staying motivated over the long term is often the hardest part of maintaining any health regimen. To keep fasting engaging, consider exploring new methods. If you've been following a particular routine, trying a different approach can reinvigorate your commitment. Perhaps you switch from daily fasting to alternate-day fasting for a month or occasionally incorporate longer fasts. This experimentation keeps fasting fresh and prevents it from becoming monotonous. Additionally, setting new goals can provide direction and achievement. Whether it's improving your metabolic markers, enhancing mental clarity, or simply feeling more energetic, having clear objectives can sustain your enthusiasm and focus.

Christina's Story: Christina began fasting in her early forties to manage her weight and energy levels. Now in her sixties, she reflects on how fasting has become a cornerstone of her health routine. She recalls how she gradually adapted her fasting schedule as her body changed, focusing more on nutrient-dense foods and mindful eating. Her commitment to fasting has helped her maintain a healthy weight, improved her mental acuity, and supported her overall well-being.

As you consider making fasting a part of your life, remember that you are not alone. Many have walked this path and found it rewarding. By embracing fasting as a flexible, evolving practice, you can enjoy its benefits for years to come. It's about creating a lifestyle that nurtures your health and enhances your quality of life, adapting as you move through different stages. Whether you're just starting or looking to deepen your commitment, fasting has the potential to be a powerful ally in your journey toward lasting wellness.

OVERCOMING OBSTACLES: STAYING MOTIVATED AND CONSISTENT

Fasting, like any lifestyle change, is not without its hurdles. For many women over forty, time management emerges as a significant challenge. Balancing fasting with busy schedules can feel overwhelming, especially when juggling work, family, and personal commitments. It's easy to feel that there aren't enough hours in the day to fit everything in. But here's a thought: View fasting not as an additional task but as a framework that simplifies your routine. By planning your fasting windows around your most hectic times, you can create space in your day. Consider aligning your fasting schedule with natural breaks, such as after morning coffee or before dinner. This way, fasting becomes a part of your routine rather than an interruption.

Here is a scenario worth considering:

Busy Morning and Evening Routine

- Your mornings are hectic with work meetings or getting the kids ready for school, so you need to focus and avoid interruptions.
- Dinner with family is a priority, and it's time to unwind after the day.

Fasting Plan Example

- Fasting window: 7 p.m.–11 a.m. (16-hour fast). This allows you to finish dinner with your family and skip breakfast the next day while still having your first meal during a natural break in the day (late morning after your meetings or tasks).

- Eating window: 11 a.m.–7 p.m. Start with a balanced, nutrient-rich meal, which fuels your day and keeps you focused. Then, have a light, healthy snack around three to keep your energy steady. Enjoy a well-balanced dinner with your family.

Benefits of This Schedule

- Creates space for uninterrupted focus during morning hours
- Allows time to enjoy dinner with family without rushing
- Maintains a balanced fasting/eating window for simplicity and sustainability

This plan prioritizes hectic times by turning fasting into a tool for productivity and calmness rather than an added stressor.

Staying motivated is another common challenge. It's normal for enthusiasm to wane, especially when results aren't immediate. Setting goals is one effective way to maintain motivation. Visualizing fasting success can be a powerful tool. Picture yourself feeling energized, wearing an outfit that makes you feel amazing, or simply enjoying a peaceful meal without distractions. These mental images can remind you about your reasons for fasting in the first place.

Alongside visualization, affirmation practices can reinforce positive mindset shifts. Each morning, take a moment to affirm your commitment to your health goals. Simple statements like "I am creating a healthier version of myself" can set a positive tone for the day. These small rituals might seem trivial, but they can significantly influence your mindset and motivation.

Consistency is the backbone of any successful fasting routine. Establishing a routine that works for you is crucial. This doesn't mean rigidly adhering to the same schedule every day but rather finding a rhythm that aligns with your lifestyle. A consistent routine helps your body adapt to fasting, making it easier to maintain over time. Consider starting with a simple schedule and gradually adjusting as you become more comfortable. Whether it's a 16:8 or a 5:2 plan, sticking to a routine can provide the structure needed to sustain your fasting practice. Over time, this consistency transforms fasting from a task into a natural part of your day.

Learning from setbacks is an invaluable part of the fasting experience. We all face disruptions—whether it's a holiday feast that throws off your schedule or a particularly stressful week that derails your plans. The key is to view these disruptions not as failures but as opportunities to build resilience.

> **Chelsey's Story:** Chelsey faced several setbacks when she began fasting. Initially, she found it challenging to maintain her schedule, often breaking her fasts earlier than planned. But rather than giving up, she used these moments to reassess and adjust her approach. She discovered that by prepping meals in advance and setting specific goals for weight loss and reducing emotional or stress-driven eating, she could better manage her fasting windows.

Resilience in fasting, much like in life, is about learning from each experience and moving forward with renewed determination. Each setback offers a chance to refine your approach, whether that means adjusting your fasting windows, trying new meal ideas, or seeking support from others. By embracing these challenges, you build the strength and confidence you need to stay committed to your fasting goals. Remember, the path to health is not a straight line but a series of steps that lead to lasting change. Each step, no matter how small, brings you closer to the radiant, healthy life you envision.

CELEBRATING SMALL WINS AND CONTINUING THE JOURNEY

Acknowledging progress is a pivotal part of any successful fasting endeavor. Each milestone, no matter how small, deserves recognition. These victories show how far you've come and reinforce the positive changes you've made. Perhaps you've managed to stick to your fasting schedule for a whole week, or maybe you've noticed a slight increase in energy during your fasting windows. Celebrate these achievements. You might set up a reward system to keep motivation high. Think of small incentives that bring you joy—perhaps a new book, a relaxing bath, or even a leisurely walk in nature. These rewards aren't just treats. They're affirmations of your hard work and commitment.

Reflection is another powerful tool in your fasting journey. Taking the time to look back on your progress fosters a deeper appreciation for your growth. Keeping a journal of successes can be an invaluable resource. Document each milestone, note the challenges you've overcome, and express how these experiences have shaped your journey. This practice highlights your achievements and provides a tangible record of your progress. When you flip through these pages, you'll see a narrative of resilience and determination—a story that's uniquely yours.

As you achieve your goals, setting new ones keeps the momentum going. Consider setting incremental goals so you build upon your previous successes. Start with something achievable, like extending your fasting window by thirty minutes or incorporating more nutrient-dense foods into your meals. These small steps pave the way for bigger accomplishments over time. With each goal met, your confidence grows, reinforcing your commitment to fasting and health. This strategy ensures continuous improvement and makes the process enjoyable and fulfilling.

Maria's Story: Maria began fasting to manage her weight

and improve her energy levels. Initially, adjusting her eating schedule was challenging, but she remained committed. Over time, she celebrated small wins, like resisting late-night snacks, and gradually worked toward her larger goals of weight loss and reducing stubborn belly fat. Maria's story is one of perseverance and dedication, illustrating how even the smallest steps can lead to significant transformations.

As you continue on this path, remember that fasting is not just about physical changes. It's a journey of personal growth and self-discovery. Embrace each moment, learn from every experience, and celebrate the progress you make along the way. Let these milestones serve as stepping stones to a healthier, more fulfilling life. As you look ahead, know that each small win brings you closer to achieving your dreams and aspirations. The journey is yours to shape, and each step forward is a testament to your strength and determination.

In recognizing these elements, you'll realize that fasting offers more than just physical benefits. It's a holistic approach that supports mental and emotional well-being, fostering empowerment and control over our health. By celebrating small wins, reflecting on your progress, and setting new goals, you create a sustainable practice that enriches your life.

CONCLUSION

"If you can see your path laid out in front of you step by step, you know it's not your path. Your own path you make with every step you take." — Joseph Campbell

As we wrap up this journey together, let's take a moment to reflect on the ground we've covered. We've explored how intermittent fasting can be a powerful tool for women over forty, especially during times of hormonal shifts that come with perimenopause, menopause, and beyond. By understanding how fasting affects hormones, you can create a personalized plan that aligns with your body's unique rhythms.

We've looked at how proper nutrition supports fasting, enhancing energy levels and mental clarity, and how these practices can lead to sustainable weight management and improved longevity.

Throughout this book, we've explored how intermittent fasting can be thoughtfully adapted to support women's health during and after their forties—a time of significant hormonal shifts and lifestyle changes. We've seen that success lies not in rigid rules but in a flexible approach that honors your body's unique needs and rhythms. Whether you've chosen to practice gentle twelve-hour fasts or found your stride with longer fasting windows, remember that this journey is deeply personal.

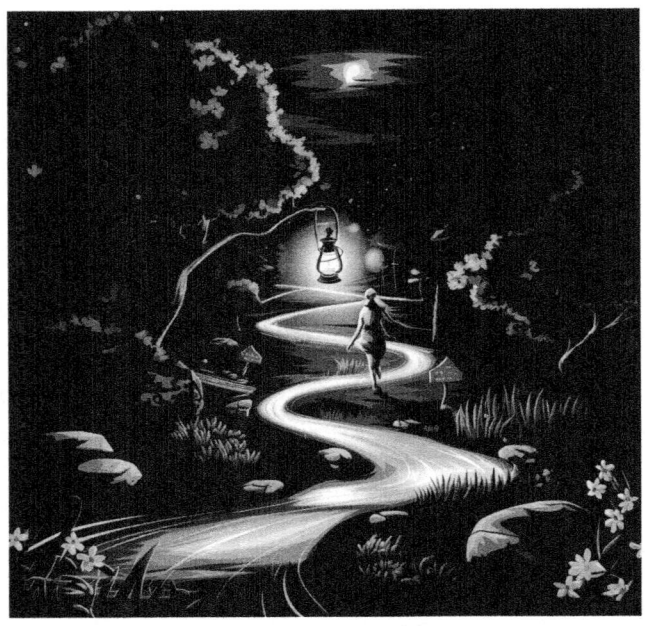

The stories shared by women in these pages demonstrate that intermittent fasting, when approached mindfully, can be more than just a weight management tool. It can be a pathway to renewed energy, mental clarity, and overall wellness.

However, the most valuable lesson remains: Listen to your body. Some days, you may feel energized during your fasting window; other days, particularly during hormonal fluctuations, you may need to adjust your approach. This adaptability isn't a sign of failure but of wisdom.

As you continue your intermittent fasting journey, carry forward the knowledge that you're not just changing when you eat—you're embracing a lifestyle that can support your health for decades to come. Stay connected with your healthcare provider, maintain awareness of your body's signals, and remember that small, consistent steps lead to lasting change. You have the power to write your own success story—one that balances the science of fasting with the art of living well in your prime years.

The purpose of this book has always been to serve as a guiding light for you, providing strategies tailored to your life stage. It's about empowering you with knowledge and practical tools to embrace fasting in a way that supports your health and well-being. Your body at forty and beyond is not a limitation; it's a powerful, adaptive ecosystem capable of remarkable resilience.

Remember, the key takeaway here is that intermittent fasting isn't about restriction or deprivation, but about strategic nourishment, hormonal balance, and holistic well-being. It's a tool for balance that helps you harmonize your body's natural processes with your lifestyle goals. It's also a compassionate approach to listening to your body, understanding its unique rhythms, and supporting its national healing mechanisms.

As you step forward, keep an open mind. Every woman's journey is unique, and what works for one may not work for another. Be gentle with yourself, and allow room for flexibility. Adapting your fasting practices as your needs change is wise and necessary. Maybe you'll find that a certain fasting schedule suits you now. But in a few months, a different approach might be better. This adaptability is a strength, not a setback.

Now, it's time to take action. You have the knowledge, tools, and confidence. The most powerful transformation happens not just in your physical body but in your mindset. Start by incorporating fasting into your daily routine and use the interactive elements we've discussed—like journaling and tracking tools—to monitor your progress. These resources are there to help you fine-tune your approach and stay motivated. Remember, change doesn't happen overnight. There will be days of remarkable success and days with challenges. Both are equally valuable. Every experiment, every adjustment, every moment of listening to your body is a step toward optimal health. With consistent effort, you'll see and feel the benefits.

There's a whole community out there waiting to support you. Engaging with others who are on similar paths can be incredibly enriching. Whether it's through online forums, social media groups, or local gatherings, connecting with others can provide encouragement and new insights. Sharing experiences and tips can make your journey less lonely and more fulfilling.

As you move forward, know that you have the power to transform your health and well-being. You are capable of incredible things. This book has given you the tools. But the real magic happens when you put them into practice. Approach your fasting journey with enthusiasm and a positive mindset. Celebrate your progress, no matter how small, and use each step as a building block for the future.

Intermittent fasting is not a destination but a lifelong journey. It will evolve as you do, and that's the beauty of it. Your needs might change tomorrow, and that's perfectly okay. Continue to explore and refine your fasting practices as you grow. Be curious and open to learning, and let this journey be one of discovery and empowerment.

Thank you for allowing me to be a part of your journey. Your commitment to your health and well-being is inspiring, and I am grateful to have shared this path with you. As you move forward, remember to embrace each step with joy and curiosity. The road ahead is full of possibilities, and you are equipped to navigate it with grace and confidence.

Here's to your health, happiness, and the exciting journey that lies ahead. May you embrace it with open arms and an open heart, knowing that each day brings new opportunities for growth and transformation.

Happy fasting!

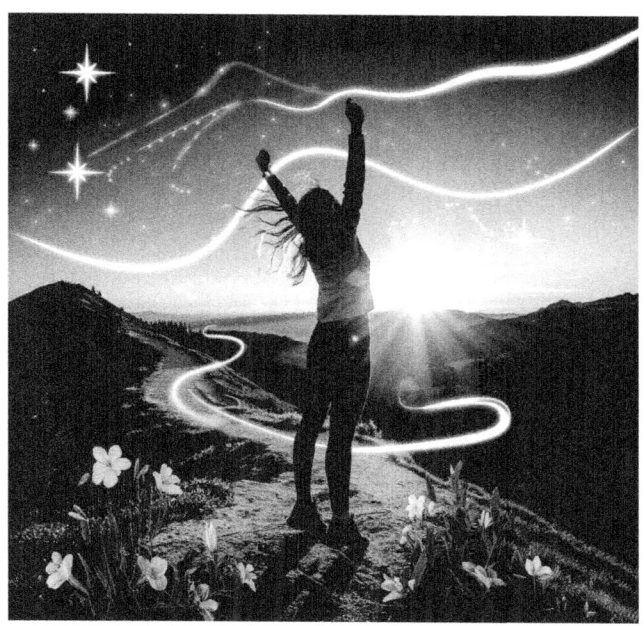

YOUR FEEDBACK MATTERS

Thank you for reading! If you enjoyed this book or found something particularly valuable in it, we would love to hear about it—and we'd be incredibly grateful for your feedback!

- What aspects of the book resonated most with you?
- Has intermittent fasting made a difference in your life?
- Were there specific chapters or sections that were particularly helpful?
- What additional information would you like to see in future resources?

Your feedback helps us and supports a community of women committed to living their best and healthy lives. Just scan the code and leave a short review.

Thank you again for choosing to read this book. Wishing you the best on your transformative journey.

Warmly,

Infinite Health Publishing

BIBLIOGRAPHY

- National Library of Medicine, "Effect of Intermittent Fasting on Reproductive Hormone Levels in Females and Males: A Review of Human Trials," https://pmc.ncbi.nlm.nih.gov/articles/PMC9182756/
- Health & Her, "Intermittent fasting for women in menopause," https://healthandher.com/en-us/blogs/expert-advice/intermittent-fasting-menopause
- National Library of Medicine, "Does Ramadan fasting has any effects on menstrual cycles?" https://pmc.ncbi.nlm.nih.gov/articles/PMC3941357/
- GlowHealth, *Intermittent Fasting Meal Plans for Women Over 40: Nourishing Your Body for Weight Loss and Hormonal Balance*, https://glowhealthco.shop/products/intermittent-fasting-meal-plans-for-women-over-40-nourishing-your-body-for-weight-loss-and-hormonal-balance
- The DUTCH Test, "Intermittent Fasting in Cycling Women: The Effects on Hormones and the Menstrual Cycle," by Jaclyn Smeaton, ND, November 18, 2022, https://dutchtest.com/blog/intermittent-fasting-in-cycling-women-the-effects-on-hormones-and-the-menstrual-cycle/
- Forbes, "Cycle Syncing: Everything You Need To Know," by Emily Laurence, last updated August 14, 2023, https://www.forbes.com/health/womens-health/cycle-syncing/
- Science Daily, "How intermittent fasting affects female hormones," October 25, 2022, https://www.sciencedaily.com/releases/2022/10/221025150257.htm
- YouTube, "Intermittent Fasting for Women," by Jason Fung ft. Megan Ramos, https://www.youtube.com/watch?v=o9YXEgMheEo
- Lose It!, "Nutrients to Keep in Mind When You're Fasting," by Kimberley Rose, RDN, CDCES, CNSC, LD, updated July 31, 2023, https://www.loseit.com/articles/nutrients-to-keep-in-mind-when-youre-fasting/
- Clem&Thyme Nutrition, "Hormone Balancing Recipes Curated by Our Dietitians," May 13, 2022, https://clemandthyme.com/2022/05/13/hormone-balancing-recipes-curated-by-our-dietitians/
- HealthLine, "Intermittent Fasting 101—The Ultimate Beginner's Guide," by Kris Gunnars, RD, updated May 3, 2024, https://www.healthline.com/nutrition/intermittent-fasting-guide

BIBLIOGRAPHY

- National Library of Medicine, "Meal Timing Regulates the Human Circadian System," https://pmc.ncbi.nlm.nih.gov/articles/PMC5483233/
- BodyLogicMD, "In Your 40s and Fatigued?" https://www.bodylogicmd.com/blog/in-your-40s-and-fatigued/#:~:text=Many%20women%20in%20their%2040s,hot%20flashes%2C%20and%20mood%20swings.&text=Thyroid%20function%20can%20change%20with,common%20as%20people%20get%20older
- Psychology Today, "Lift Up Your Eating Energy With Intermittent Fasting," by Michael J. Breus, PhD, March 1, 2022, https://www.psychologytoday.com/us/blog/sleep-newzzz/202203/lift-up-your-eating-energy-with-intermittent-fasting
- HealthLine, "Best Foods to Boost Your Brain and Memory," https://www.healthline.com/nutrition/11-brain-foods
- Zero Longevity, "How to Pair Mindful Eating with Mindful Fasting," Nichole Grant, RD, August 21, 2023, https://zerolongevity.com/blog/how-to-pair-mindful-eating-with-mindful-fasting/#:~:text=The%20term%20%E2%80%9Cmindful%20fasting%E2%80%9D%20can,responses%20during%20the%20fasting%20process
- Everyday Health, "What Midlife Women Should Know About Intermittent Fasting," Meryl Davids Landau, updated January 4, 2023, https://www.everydayhealth.com/womens-health/what-midlife-women-should-know-about-intermittent-fasting/
- BodyLogicMD, "Tips for Balancing Hormones and Wellness for Women Over 40," https://www.bodylogicmd.com/blog/womens-age-40-wellness-tip-hormone-balance/
- Physicians Committee for Responsible Medicine, "Fighting Hot Flashes With Diet," https://www.pcrm.org/clinical-research/fighting-hot-flashes-with-diet
- Harvard Health Publishing, "Omega-3 fatty acids for mood disorders," by David Mischoulon, MD, PhD, October 27, 2020, https://www.health.harvard.edu/blog/omega-3-fatty-acids-for-mood-disorders-2018080314414
- National Library of Medicine, "Intermittent and periodic fasting, longevity and disease," https://pmc.ncbi.nlm.nih.gov/articles/PMC8932957/
- Science Direct, "The effect of prolonged intermittent fasting on autophagy, inflammasome, and senescence genes expressions: An exploratory study in healthy young males," https://www.sciencedirect.com/science/article/pii/S2666149723000063

BIBLIOGRAPHY

- Mayo Clinic, "Fasting diet: Can it improve my heart health?" by Donald Hensrud, MD, https://www.mayoclinic.org/diseases-conditions/heart-disease/expert-answers/fasting-diet/faq-20058334#:~:text=Some%20studies%20say%20that%20intermittent,helps%20control%20blood%20sugar%20levels
- Diabetes Voice, "The benefits of fasting for diabetes management and prevention," by Justine Evans, March 8, 2024, https://diabetesvoice.org/en/caring-for-diabetes/the-benefits-of-fasting-for-diabetes-management-and-prevention/
- Dr. Margaretha Montagu, "Journaling Prompts for Women on a Weight Loss Mission," https://margarethamontagu.com/writing-meditation-for-intermittent-fasters-journaling-prompts-for-women-on-a-weight-loss-mission/
- Healthline, "Intermittent Fasting For Women: A Beginner's Guide" https://www.healthline.com/nutrition/intermittent-fasting-for-women
- North East Islamic Community Center, "What Are the Benefits of Fasting for the Society?" https://islamiccenter.org/what-are-the-benefits-of-fasting-for-the-society/
- BodyFast, "How to Reconcile Intermittent Fasting With Your Family Life," https://www.bodyfast.app/en/fasting-and-family-life/
- Indeed for Employers, "An Employer's Guide to Fasting at Work: What to Expect and How to Support Employees," https://www.indeed.com/hire/c/info/fasting-at-work
- Lifesum, "How to Navigate Social Situations While Fasting," August 16, 2023, https://lifesum.com/nutrition-explained/how-to-navigate-social-situations-while-fasting
- WebMD, "Intermittent Fasting for Women Over 50: What You Need to Know," by Stephanie Booth, https://www.webmd.com/healthy-aging/what-to-know-about-intermittent-fasting-for-women-after-50

Printed in Dunstable, United Kingdom

64992474R00080